Reflux Laryngitis
and Related Disorders

Reflux Laryngitis and Related Disorders

Robert T. Sataloff, M.D., D.M.A.
Professor of Otolaryngology—Head and Neck Surgery
Department of Otolaryngology—Head and Neck Surgery
Thomas Jefferson University
Chairman, Department of Otolaryngology—Head and Neck Surgery
Graduate Hospital
Adjunct Professor of Otorhinolaryngology
University of Pennsylvania
Adjunct Professor of Otolaryngology—Head and Neck Surgery
Georgetown University
Chairman, Board of Directors
The Voice Foundation
Chairman, American Institute for Voice and Ear Research
Philadelphia, Pennsylvania

Donald O. Castell, M.D.
Kimbel Professor and Chairman
Department of Medicine
Graduate Hospital
Philadelphia, Pennsylvania

Philip O. Katz, M.D.
Director, Comprehensive Chest Pain and Swallowing Center
Graduate Hospital
Philadelphia, Pennsylvania

Dahlia M. Sataloff, M.D., F.A.C.S.
Associate Professor of Surgery
Medical College of Pennsylvania/Hahnemann School of Medicine
Attending Surgeon
Graduate Hospital
Philadelphia, Pennsylvania

SINGULAR PUBLISHING GROUP, INC
SAN DIEGO · LONDON

Notice: The indications, procedures, drug dosages, and diagnosis and remediation protocols in this book have been recommended in the clinical literature and conform to the practices of the general medical and health services communities. All procedures put forth in this book should be performed only by trained, licensed practitioners. The diagnostic and remediation protocols and the medications described do not necessarily have specific approval by the Food And Drug Administration for use in the disorders and/or diseases and dosages for which they are recommended. Because standards of practice and usage change, it is the responsibility of practitioners to keep abreast of revised recommendations, dosages, and procedures.

Singular Publishing Group, Inc.
401 West A Street, Suite 325
San Diego, California 92101-7904

Singular Publishing Ltd.
19 Compton Terrace
London N1 2UN, UK

Singular Publishing Group, Inc., publishes textbooks, clinical manuals, clinical reference books, journals, videos, and multimedia materials on speech-language pathology, audiology, otorhinolaryngology, special education, early childhood, aging, occupational therapy, physical therapy, rehabilitation, counseling, mental health, and voice. For your convenience, our entire catalog can be accessed on our website at *http://www.singpub.com*. Our mission to provide you with materials to meet the daily challenges of the ever-changing health care/educational environment will remain on course if we are in touch with you. In that spirit, we welcome your feedback on our products. Please telephone (**1-800-521-8545**), fax (**1-800-774-8398**), or e-mail (*singpub@singpub.com*) your comments and requests to us.

© 1999, by Singular Publishing Group, Inc.

Typeset in 10/12 Palatino by Thompson Type
Printed in the United States of America by McNaughton and Gunn

All rights, including that of translation, reserved. No part of this publication may be reproduced, stored in a retrieval system or transmitted in any form or by any means, electronic, mechanical, recording, or otherwise, without prior written permission of the publisher.

Library of Congress Cataloging-in-Publication Data

Reflux laryngitis and related disorders / by Robert T. Sataloff . . . [et al.].
    p. cm.
   Includes bibliographical references and index.
   ISBN 0-7693-0014-6 (softcover : alk. paper)
   1. Laryngitis--Etiology. 2. Gastroesophageal reflux--Complications.
3. Laryngitis--Treatment. 4. Gastroesophageal reflux--Treatment. I. Sataloff, Robert Thayer.
   [DNLM: 1. Laryngitis--etiology. 2. Laryngitis--diagnosis.
3. Gastroesophageal   Reflux--complications. 4. Gastroesophageal Reflux--therapy.   WV 510 R332 1999]
RF520.R44   1999
616.2'2071--DC21
DNLM/DLC
for Library of Congress   98-49305
                                                                                 CIP

Contents

	Preface	vii
	About the Authors	ix
1	Introduction	1
2	Anatomy and Physiology of the Voice	5
3	Anatomy and Physiology of the Esophagus and Its Sphincters	19
4	Gastroesophageal Reflux Disease: An Overview of Clinical Presentation and Epidemiology	33
5	Reflux Laryngitis and Other Otolaryngologic Manifestations of Laryngopharyngeal Reflux	41
6	Diagnostic Tests for Gastroesophageal Reflux	55
7	Behavioral and Medical Management of Gastroesophageal Reflux Disease	69
8	Surgical Therapy for Gastroesophageal Reflux Disease	89
	Index	107

Preface

Reflux laryngitis is an extremely common condition that is often overlooked. Because patients with reflux laryngitis and other symptoms and signs of laryngopharyngeal reflux often do not complain of heartburn, many patients and their physicians do not recognize that their symptoms are being caused by gastroesophageal reflux disease. Because reflux is so frequently responsible for hoarseness, halitosis, symptoms of "postnasal drip," recurrent sore throat, chronic cough, reactive airway symptoms, and other common maladies, it is useful for all healthcare providers to be familiar with reflux laryngitis and related disorders. Such familiarity is especially important because untreated reflux may lead to Barrett's esophagus and to carcinoma of the esophagus or larynx.

This book is intended to provide a practical overview of reflux laryngitis and other manifestations of laryngopharyngeal reflux. It is designed for use by otolaryngologists, primary care physicians, internists, gastroenterologists, general surgeons, speech-language pathologists, voice teachers, and patients. Chapter 1 introduces laryngopharyngeal reflux as a multi-system disorder and its importance in otolaryngologic and pulmonary conditions. Chapter 2 summarizes the complex structure and function of the human voice, laying the scientific groundwork necessary to understand the ways in which reflux can impair voice use. Chapter 3 defines esophageal structure and functions, providing a comprehensive review of the mechanisms of swallowing and a concise discussion of the physiology of the lower esophageal sphincter. Chapter 4 reviews the symptoms associated with not only typical gastroesophageal reflux disease, but also with atypical (extra-esophageal) reflux, including laryngopharyngeal reflux complaints and other symptoms such as chest pain. This chapter also reviews complications of reflux such as Barrett's esophagus.

Chapter 5 provides a comprehensive discussion of laryngopharyngeal reflux and the symptoms and signs associated with peptic mucositis of the larynx and related structures. This chapter also reviews much of the literature on reflux laryngitis and stresses some particularly important reflux-related conditions such as laryngeal granuloma. Chapter 6 reviews the diagostic tests available for patients with suspected reflux and the uses, strengths, and shortcomings of each procedure. Chapter 7 reviews the latest concepts in medical and behavioral management of reflux disease. Chapter 8 describes surgery for reflux, including an in-depth explanation of laparoscopic antireflux surgery, clearly illustrated by surgeon-medical illustrator John Potochny, M.D.

In an effort to make this book useful for health care providers and reflux sufferers, we have tried to keep this text clear and concise. It is our hope that the book will increase awareness of laryngopharyngeal reflux and its importance in clinical practice.

Robert Thayer Sataloff, M.D., D.M.A.
Donald O. Castell, M.D.
Philip O. Katz, M.D.
Dahlia M. Sataloff, M.D., F.A.C.S.

About the Authors

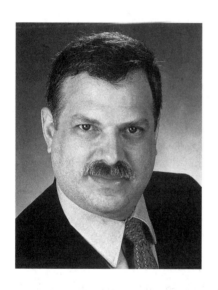

Robert T. Sataloff, M.D., D.M.A.
Dr. Sataloff is Professor of Otolaryngology—Head and Neck Surgery at Jefferson Medical College, Thomas Jefferson University; Chairman of the Department of Otolaryngology—Head and Neck Surgery of Graduate Hospital; Adjunct Professor of Otorhinolaryngology, University of Pennsylvania, Department of Otolaryngology—Head and Neck Surgery; and Adjunct Professor of Otolaryngology—Head and Neck Surgery at Georgetown University; on the faculties of the Academy of Vocal Arts and the Curtis Institute of Music; Conductor of the Thomas Jefferson University Choir and Orchestra; Director of the Jefferson Arts Medicine Center; and Chairman of the Board of Directors of the Voice Foundation and the American Institute for Voice and Ear Research. Dr. Sataloff is also a professional singer and singing teacher. He holds an undergraduate degree from Haverford College in Music Theory and Composition, a medical degree from Jefferson Medical College, received a Doctor of Musical Arts in Voice Performance from Combs College of Music, and completed his residency in Otolaryngology—Head and Neck Surgery at the University of Michigan. He also completed a Fellowship in Otology, Neurotology, and Skull Base Surgery at the University of Michigan. He is Editor-in-Chief of the *Journal of Voice*, Editor-in-Chief of the *Journal of Occupational Hearing Loss*, on the Editorial Boards of the *Journal of Singing*, *Medical Problems of Performing*

Artists, and *Ear, Nose & Throat Journal*, and serves on the Editorial Review Boards of many major otolaryngology journals in the United States. Dr. Sataloff has written over 400 publications, including 17 textbooks. His medical practice is limited to care of the professional voice and to neurotology-skull base surgery.

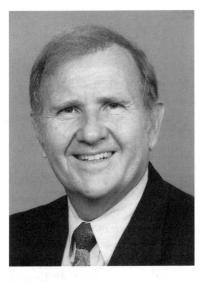

Donald O. Castell, M.D.
Kimbel Professor and Chairman
Department of Medicine
Graduate Hospital
Philadelphia, Pennsylvania

Donald Castell, M.D., is a 1960 graduate of the George Washington University School of Medicine and served as a medical officer in the U.S. Navy from 1959 to 1979. Before retiring with the rank of captain, he spent his last 4 years of active service as Chairman of Medicine at the National Naval Medical Center at Bethesda, Maryland. He has held faculty positions at George Washington University School of Medicine, the Uniformed Services University of Health Sciences, Bowman Gray School of Medicine in Winston-Salem, North Carolina, and Jefferson Medical College in Philadelphia, Pennsylvania. Since April 1992, he has been in his current position of Kimbel Professor and Chairman of the Department of Medicine at Graduate Hospital in Philadelphia, Pennsylvania.

Dr. Castell is internationally recognized as a leading authority on diseases of the esophagus and esophageal function and has authored or co-authored more than 500 scientific publications. He is also the editor and principal contributor of *The Esophagus,* the primary text on this subject, a definitive 842-page text published by Little, Brown, and Company.

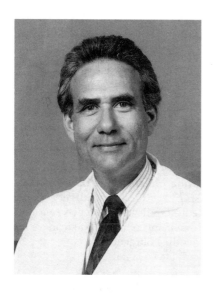

Philip O. Katz, M.D.
Director, Comprehensive Chest Pain
 and Swallowing Center
Vice Chairman, Department of
 Medicine
Graduate Hospital
Philadelphia, Pennsylvania

In 1978, Dr. Katz received his medical degree from Bowman Gray School of Medicine, Wake Forest University, Winston-Salem, North Carolina. He served his residency and chief residency in internal medicine, followed by a fellowship in gastroenterology, at the Bowman Gray School of Medicine. He completed a faculty development fellowship at The Johns Hopkins University, Baltimore, Maryland. He is board-certified in internal medicine and gastroenterology.

Dr. Katz is a fellow of the American College of Physicians and the American College of Gastroenterology. He has served as Chairman of the Educational Affairs Committee of the American College of Gastroenterology since 1996. Dr. Katz participates in numerous other national and local organizations such as the American Gastroenterology Association and The American Society of Gastrointestinal Endoscopy. Dr. Katz has contributed to the publication of 60 papers, abstracts, monographs, and book chapters.

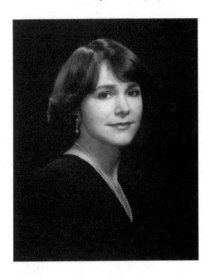

Dahlia M. Sataloff, M.D.
Associate Professor of Surgery
Medical College of Pennsylvania/
Hahnemann School of Medicine
Attending Surgeon
Graduate Hospital

Dahlia M. Sataloff, M.D., F.A.C.S., matriculated cum laude from the University of Michigan Medical School. Having completed her residency in general surgery at Pennsylvania Hospital in Philadelphia, she is currently staff attending surgeon at Pennsylvania Hospital and Graduate Hospital and Associate Professor of Surgery at the Medical College of Pennsylvania/Hahnemann School of Medicine.

DEDICATION

This book is dedicated to Ben and John Sataloff,
June Castell, and Leilani Eveland

CHAPTER 1

Introduction

Laryngopharyngeal reflux (LPR) is a form of gastro-esophageal reflux disease (GERD). Reflux laryngitis (RL) is only one component of LPR. Usually, when RL is present, symptoms and signs of more generalized LPR are also present, although they are commonly missed if not elicited by specific questions during the medical history.

Occult chronic gastroesophageal reflux is an etiologic factor in a high percentage of patients with laryngological (ie, voice) complaints. Although it is seen in otolaryngologic patients of all ages, the problem appears to be particularly common in professional voice users and singers. In 1991, Sataloff et al reported reflux laryngitis in 265 of 583 consecutive professional voice users (45%), including singers and others, who sought medical care during a 12-month period, although reflux laryngitis was often diagnosed incidentally and was not always responsible for the patient's primary voice complaint.[1] The incidence may be lower in patients with other vocations, but it is interesting to note that Koufman et al found increased gastroesophageal reflux in 78% of patients with hoarseness[2] and in about 50% of all patients with voice complaints (J.A. Koufman, personal communication, October 1995). Nevertheless, additional studies of the epidemiology and prevalence of reflux laryngitis are needed to help clarify the clinical importance of this entity.

LPR is a multi-system disorder. It involves the sphincter between the stomach and distal esophagus; the entire length of the esophagus; the upper esophageal sphincter; the structures of the larynx, pharynx, and oral cavity; and the trachea and lungs. Consequently, it should be evident that LPR is managed best through a team approach. The team includes at least a laryngologist, gastroenterologist, GI (gastrointestinal) laboratory personnel, speech-language pathologist, and pulmonologist. For voice professionals, a singing voice specialist and an acting voice specialist should be included.[3] The availability of a knowledgeable psychologist and nutritionist is highly desirable, as well.[3,4] Although it is possible for one physician to manage most or all aspects of LPR, this approach does not provide comprehensive state-of-the-art care. The laryngologist is uniquely qualified to diagnose disorders of the larynx. Laryngeal involvement commonly results in dysphonia for which patients attempt to compensate through hyperfunctional voice use patterns (muscular tension dysphonia [MTD]). The collaboration of a speech-language pathologist and other voice team members is invaluable in eliminating compensatory behaviors and optimizing phonatory technique. Although laryngologists can certainly purchase 24-hour pH monitoring equipment and may even perform manometry, they do not generally do so with the same level of expertise as a gastroenterologist whose entire career is devoted to disorders of the esophagus. Just as certain laryngologists subspecialize in voice care, some gastroenterologists subspecialize in the management of reflux. This group of professionals and their ancillary staff are best equipped to diagnose and treat reflux and its consequences. Laryngopharyngeal reflux is almost always associated with some degree of aspiration. This may be clinically insignificant, or it may cause chronic cough, reactive airway disease, difficulties controlling asthma, pneumonia, or bronchiectasis. A knowledgeable pulmonologist is essential in recognizing and treating these conditions.

There are several issues of special concern in the management of otolaryngologic patients with reflux, especially professional voice users who require particularly good control of reflux disease. First, many of these patients are young and will require prolonged or lifetime use of high doses of H_2 antagonists or proton pump inhibitors. The long-term effects of these medications are unknown, and they are expensive. The cost may be burdensome to performers, and a financial strain often leads to poor compliance. Second, in general, medications do not cure reflux. They simply neutralize the refluxate, but they effectively control symptoms in many patients. However, some patients may continue to aspirate pH-neutral fluid, bile salts, and other substances not appropriate for entry into the pharynx, larynx, and lungs. In professional singers and other high-performance vocalists, this problem may continue to be symptomatic (throat clearing, excess phlegm, cough) even when acidity is well controlled, although no one has demonstrated that de-acidified gastric juice actually causes mucosal injury. Conveniently, surgical therapy for GERD has improved dramatically with the advent of laparoscopic Nissen fundoplication, making both chronic medical or surgical therapy good options for consideration by the patient. An increasing percentage of patients is being referred for surgery. It is essential for otolaryngologists to be familiar with the anatomy, physiology, pathology, diagnosis, and treatment options for LPR and GERD in general. Although much of this knowledge is outside traditional otolaryngology training and is not intended to make the otolaryngologist an amateur gastroenterologist, familiarity with the latest concepts and techniques helps the otolaryngologist assemble an appropriate team, guide its management of voice patients, interpret information from other colleagues on the reflux care team in the light of laryngologic symptoms and needs, and assure optimal patient care.

REFERENCES

1. Sataloff RT, Spiegel JR, Hawkshaw MJ. Strobovideolaryngoscopy: results and clinical value. *Ann Otol Rhinol Laryngol.* 1991;100:725–727.
2. Koufman JA, Wiener GJ, Wu WC, Castell DO. Reflux laryngitis and its sequelae: the diagnostic role of ambulatory 24-hour pH monitoring. *J Voice.* 1988;2:78–89.
3. Sataloff RT. *Professional Voice: The Science and Art of Clinical Care.* 2nd ed. San Diego, Calif: Singular Publishing Group; 1997:1–1069.
4. Rosen DC, Sataloff RT: *The Psychology of Voice Disorders.* San Diego, Calif: Singular Publishing Group; 1997:1–284.

CHAPTER 2

Anatomy and Physiology of the Voice

The anatomic and physiologic basis for many symptoms of LPR is fairly obvious. Topical irritation, muscle spasm, and bronchospasm in response to acidic aspiration, halitosis, sore throat, and other symptoms are easy to understand, although some have unexpectedly complex physiology. However, the effects of reflux laryngitis on voice function are often greater than one might anticipate based on physical findings. To understand the impact of reflux disease on phonation, it is helpful to review current concepts in anatomy and physiology of the voice. Naturally, the physiology of phonation is much more complex than this brief chapter might imply. Readers interested in acquiring more than a clinically essential introduction are encouraged to consult other literature, including Sundberg's excellent text *The Science of the Singing Voice*,[1] an overview of the mechanics of phonation, by Scherer,[2] selected chapters in Sataloff's *Professional Voice: The Science and Art of Clinical Care (2nd ed.)*,[3] and the numerous references and suggested readings compiled in these sources.

ANATOMY

The *larynx* is essential to normal voice production, but the anatomy of the voice is not limited to the larynx. The vocal mechanism includes the abdominal and back musculature, rib cage, lungs, and the pharynx, oral cavity, and nose. Each component performs an important function in voice production, although it is possible to produce voice even without a larynx, for example, in patients who have undergone laryngectomy. In addition, virtually all parts of the body play some role in voice production and may contribute to voice dysfunction. Even something as remote as a sprained ankle may alter posture, thereby impairing abdominal, back, and thoracic muscle function and resulting in vocal inefficiency, weakness, and hoarseness.

The larynx is composed of 4 basic anatomic units: the skeleton, intrinsic muscles, extrinsic muscles and mucosa. The most important parts of the laryngeal skeleton are the thyroid cartilage, cricoid cartilage, and two arytenoid cartilages (Fig 2-1). Intrinsic muscles of the larynx are connected to these cartilages (Fig 2-2). One of the intrinsic muscles, the *thyroarytenoid* or *vocalis muscle*, extends on each side from the arytenoid cartilage to the inside of the thyroid cartilage just below and behind the "Adam's apple," forming the body of the vocal folds (popularly called the vocal cords). The vocal folds act as the *oscillator* or *voice source* of the vocal tract. The space between the vocal folds is called the *glottis* and is used as an anatomic reference point. The intrinsic muscles alter the position, shape, and tension of the vocal folds, bringing them together (adduction), apart (abduction), or stretching them by increasing longitudinal tension (Fig 2-3). They are able to do so because the laryngeal cartilages are connected by soft attachments that allow changes in their relative angles and distances, thereby permitting alteration in the shape and tension of the tissues suspended between them. The arytenoids are also capable of rocking, rotating, and gliding, permitting complex vocal fold motion and alteration in the shape of the vocal fold edge (Fig 2-4). All but one of the muscles on each side of the larynx are innervated by 1 of the 2 recurrent laryngeal nerves. Because this structure runs a long course from the neck down into the chest and then back up to the larynx (hence, the name "recurrent"), it is easily injured by trauma, neck surgery, and chest surgery, which may result in vocal fold paralysis. The remaining muscle (*cricothyroid muscle*) is innervated by the *superior laryngeal nerve* on each side, which is especially susceptible to viral and traumatic injury. It produces increases in longitudinal tension that are important in volume and pitch control. The "false vocal folds" are located above the vocal folds and, unlike the true vocal folds, do not make contact during normal speaking or singing. The neuroanatomy and neurophysiology of phonation are exceedingly complicated and only partially understood. As the new field of neurolaryngology advances, a more thorough understanding of the subject will become increasingly important to clinicians. Readers interested in acquiring a deeper, scientific understanding are encouraged to consult the growing literature

Anatomy and Physiology of the Voice

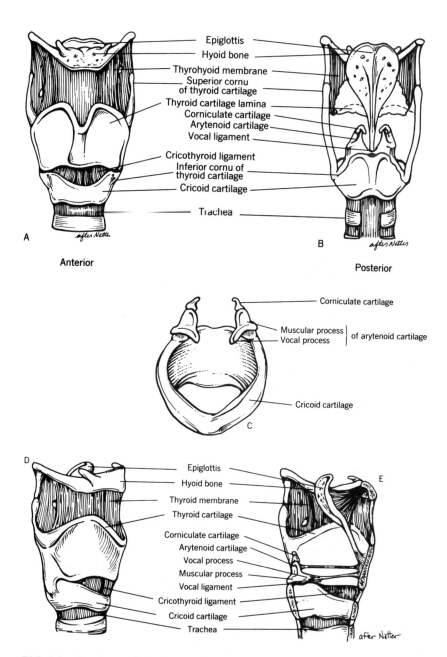

FIG 2-1. Cartilages of the larynx. (From Sataloff R, *Professional Voice: The Science and Art of Clinical Care.* 2 ed. San Diego: Singular Pubishing Group; 1997:112, with permission.)

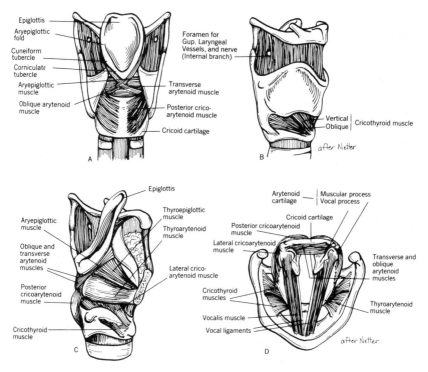

FIG 2-2. Intrinsic muscles of the larynx. (From Sataloff R, *Professional Voice: The Science and Art of Clinical Care.* 2 ed. San Diego: Singular Publishing Group; 1997:118, with permission.)

on this subject, particularly a fine, well referenced review by Garrett and Larson.[4]

Because the attachments of the laryngeal cartilages are flexible, the positions of the cartilages with respect to each other change when the laryngeal skeleton is elevated or lowered. Such changes in vertical height are controlled by the extrinsic laryngeal muscles, or strap muscles, of the neck. When the angles and distances between the cartilages change because of this accordion effect, the resting length of the intrinsic muscles is changed as a consequence. Such large adjustments in intrinsic muscle condition interfere with fine control of smooth vocal quality. This is why classically trained singers are generally taught to use their extrinsic muscles to maintain the laryngeal skeleton at a relatively constant height, regardless of pitch. That is, they learn to avoid the natural tendency of the larynx to rise with ascending pitch and fall with descending pitch, thereby enhancing unity of quality throughout the vocal range.

Anatomy and Physiology of the Voice

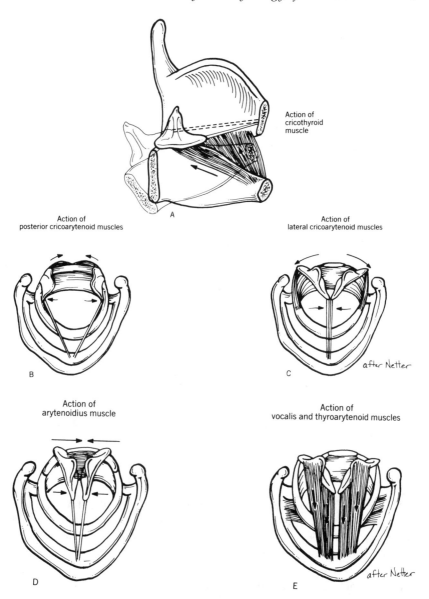

FIG 2-3. Action of the intrinsic muscles. (From Sataloff R, *Professional Voice: The Science and Art of Clinical Care.* 2 ed. San Diego: Singular Publishing Group; 1997:119, with permission.)

The soft tissues lining the larynx are much more complex than originally thought. The mucosa forms the thin, lubricated surface of the vocal folds that makes contact when the two vocal folds are closed.

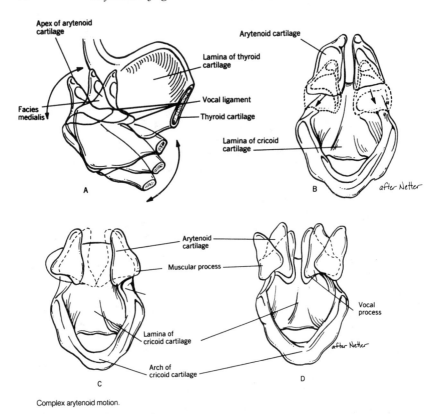

FIG 2-4. Complex arytenoid motion. (From Gould WJ, Sataloff RT, Spiegel JR. *Voice Surgery.* St Louis, Mo: Mosby-Yearbook; 1993:164.)

It looks like the mucosa lining the inside of the mouth. Throughout most of the larynx, there are goblet cells and pseudo-stratified ciliated columnar epithelium designed for handling mucous secretions, similar to mucosa found throughout the respiratory tract. However, the mucosa overlying the vocal folds is different. First, it is stratified squamous epithelium, better suited to withstand the trauma of vocal fold contact. Second, the vocal fold is not simply muscle covered with mucosa. Rather, as described by Hirano,[5] it consists of 5 layers. Mechanically, the vocal fold structures act more like 3 layers, consisting of the *cover* (epithelium and superficial layer of the lamina propria), *transition* (intermediate and deep layers of the lamina propria), and *body* (the vocalis muscle). Surgeons must understand this anatomy and the importance of preserving it during surgical intervention.

The *supraglottic vocal tract* includes the pharynx, tongue, palate, oral cavity, nose, and other structures. Together, they act as a *resonator* and are largely responsible for vocal quality or timbre and the perceived character of all speech sounds. The vocal folds themselves produce only a "buzzing" sound. During the course of vocal training for singing, acting, or healthy speaking, changes occur not only in the larynx, but also in the muscle motion, control, and shape of the supraglottic vocal tract.

The *infraglottic vocal tract* serves as the *power source* for the voice. Singers and actors refer to the entire power source complex as their "support" or "diaphragm." Actually, the anatomy of support for phonation is especially complicated and not completely understood. Yet, it is quite important because deficiencies in support are frequently responsible for voice dysfunction.

The purpose of the support mechanism is to generate a force that directs a controlled airstream between the vocal folds. Active respiratory muscles work in concert with passive forces. The principal muscles of inspiration are the diaphragm (a dome-shaped muscle that extends along the bottom of the rib cage) and the external intercostal muscles. During quiet respiration, expiration is largely passive. The lungs and rib cage generate passive expiratory forces under many common circumstances such as after a full breath.

Many of the muscles used for active expiration are also employed in "support" for phonation. Muscles of active expiration either raise the intra-abdominal pressure, forcing the diaphragm upward, or lower the ribs or sternum to decrease the dimensions of the thorax, or both, thereby compressing air in the chest. The primary muscles of expiration are "the abdominal muscles," but the internal intercostals and other chest and back muscles are also involved. Trauma or surgery that alters the structure or function of these muscles or ribs undermines the power source of the voice as do diseases that impair expiration, such as asthma. Deficiencies in the support mechanism often result in compensatory efforts that utilize the laryngeal muscles, which are not designed for power source functions. Such behavior can result in decreased function, rapid voice fatigue, pain and even structural pathology including vocal fold nodules.

PHYSIOLOGY OF THE VOICE

The physiology of voice production is complex. Volitional production of voice begins in the cerebral cortex (Fig 2-5). The command for vocalization involves interaction among centers for speech and other areas

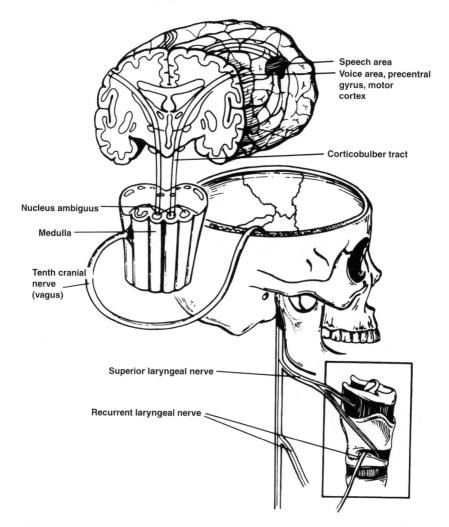

FIG 2-5. Simplified summary of pathway for volitional phonation. (From Gould WJ, Sataloff RT, Spiegel JR. *Voice Surgery*. St. Louis, Mo: Mosby-Yearbook; 1993:166, with permission.)

of the brain. For singing, speech directives must be integrated with information from the brain centers for musical and artistic expression. The "idea" of the planned vocalization is conveyed to the precentral gyrus in the motor cortex, which transmits another set of instructions to the motor nuclei in the brain stem and spinal cord. These areas send out the complicated messages necessary for coordinated activity of the larynx, thoracic and abdominal musculature, and vocal tract articulators. Additional refinement of motor activity is provided by the extrapyramidal and autonomic nervous systems. These impulses combine to produce a sound that is transmitted not only to the ears of the listener, but also to those of the speaker or singer. Auditory feedback is transmitted from the ear through the brain stem to the cerebral cortex, and adjustments are made to permit the vocalist to match the sound produced with the sound intended, taking into account the acoustic properties of the environment. There is also tactile feedback from the throat and muscles involved in phonation that is believed to help in the fine tuning of vocal output, although the mechanism and role of tactile feedback are not fully understood. In many trained singers and speakers, the ability to use tactile feedback effectively is cultivated because of expected interference with auditory feedback by ancillary noise such as an orchestra or band.

Phonation requires interaction among the power source, oscillator, and resonator. The voice may be likened to a brass instrument such as a trumpet. Power is generated by the chest, abdomen, and back musculature, producing a high-pressure airstream. The trumpeter's lips open and close against the mouthpiece, producing a buzz similar to the sound produced by the vocal folds. This sound then passes through the trumpet, which has resonance characteristics that shape the sound we associate with trumpet music. The nonmouthpiece portion of a brass instrument is analogous to the supraglottic vocal tract.

During phonation, rapid, complex adjustments of the infraglottic musculature are necessary because the resistance changes almost continuously as the glottis closes, opens and changes shape. At the beginning of each phonatory cycle, the vocal folds are approximated. That is, the glottis is obliterated. This permits infraglottic pressure to build up, typically to a level of about 7 cm of water for conversational speech. At this point, the vocal folds are convergent (Fig 2-6.1). Because the vocal folds are closed, there is no airflow. The subglottic pressure pushes the vocal folds progressively further apart from the bottom up (Figs 2-6.1 and 2-6.2) until a space develops (Fig 2-6.3) and air begins to flow. Bernoulli force created by the air passes between the vocal folds and combines with the mechanical properties of the folds to begin closing the lower portion of the glottis almost immediately (Figs 2-6.4, 2-6.5, 2-6.6, and 2-6.7) even while the upper edges are still separating. The upper portion of the vocal folds has strong elastic properties, which tend to make the vocal folds snap back to the midline. This force becomes more dominant as the upper edges are stretched farther apart, and as the force of the air stream diminishes because of approximation of the lower edges of the vocal folds. Therefore, the upper portions of the vocal folds return to the midline (Fig 2-6.8 and 2-6.9) completing the glottic cycle. Subglottal pressure then builds again (Fig 2-6.10), and

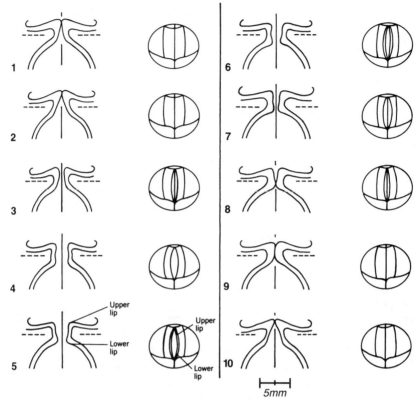

FIG 2-6. Frontal view (*left*) and view from above (*right*) illustrating the normal pattern of vocal fold vibration. The vocal folds close and open the glottis from the inferior aspect of the vibratory margin upwards. (From Hirano M, *Clinical Examination of the Voice.* New York: Springer-Verlag; 1981:44, with permission.)

the events are repeated. The frequency of vibration (number of cycles of openings and closings per second, measured in hertz [Hz]) is dependent on the air pressure and mechanical properties of the vocal folds, which are regulated by the laryngeal muscles.

Frequency corresponds closely with our perception of pitch. Under most circumstances, as the vocal folds are thinned and stretched, and air pressure is increased, the frequency of air pulse emission increases, and pitch goes up. In understanding this myoelastic-aerodynamic mechanism of phonation, it is important to note that the vocal folds not only emit pulses of air rather than vibrating like strings, but that there also is a vertical phase difference. That is, the lower portion of the vocal folds begins to open and close before the upper portion. The rippling displacement of the vocal fold cover produces a mucosal wave that can be examined clinically under stroboscopic light. If this complex motion is impaired, hoarseness or other changes in voice quality may result.

The sound produced by the vibrating vocal folds (voice source signal) is a complex tone containing a fundamental frequency and many overtones, or higher harmonic partials. The amplitude of the partials decreases uniformly at approximately 12 dB per octave. Interestingly, the spectrum of the voice source is about the same in ordinary speakers as it is in singers and trained speakers. However, voice quality differences occur as the voice source signal passes through the supraglottic vocal tract (Fig 2-7).

The pharynx, oral cavity, and nasal cavity act as a series of interconnected resonators, more complex than a trumpet or other single resonators. As with other resonators, some frequencies are attenuated, others are enhanced. Enhanced frequencies are radiated with higher relative amplitudes. Sundberg has shown that the vocal tract has 4 or 5 important resonance frequencies called formants.[1] The presence of formants alters the uniformly sloping voice source spectrum, creating peaks at formant frequencies. These alterations of the voice source spectral envelope are responsible for distinguishable sounds of speech and song. Formant frequencies are established by vocal tract shape, which can be altered by laryngeal, pharyngeal, and oral cavity musculature. While overall vocal tract length and shape are individually fixed and determined by age and sex (females and children have shorter vocal tracts and formant frequencies that are higher than males), mastering adjustment of vocal tract shape is fundamental to voice training. Although the formants differ for different vowels, one resonant frequency, known as the "singer's formant," has received particular attention. The singer's formant occurs in the vicinity of 2300 Hz to 3200 Hz for all vowel spectra and appears to be responsible for the "ring" in a singer's or trained speaker's voice. The ability to hear a trained voice clearly even over a loud choir or orchestra is dependent primarily on the presence of the singer's formant.[1] Interestingly, there is little or no significant difference in maximum vocal intensity between a trained and an untrained singer. The singer's formant also contributes significantly to the difference in timbre among voice categories, occurring in basses at about 2400 Hz, baritones at 2600 Hz, tenors at 2800 Hz, mezzo-sopranos at 2900 Hz, and sopranos at 3200 Hz. It is much less prominent in high soprano singing.

Control mechanisms for 2 vocal characteristics, fundamental frequency and intensity, are particularly important. Fundamental frequency, which corresponds to pitch, can be altered by changing either the air pressure or the mechanical properties of the vocal folds, although the latter is more efficient under most conditions. Contracting

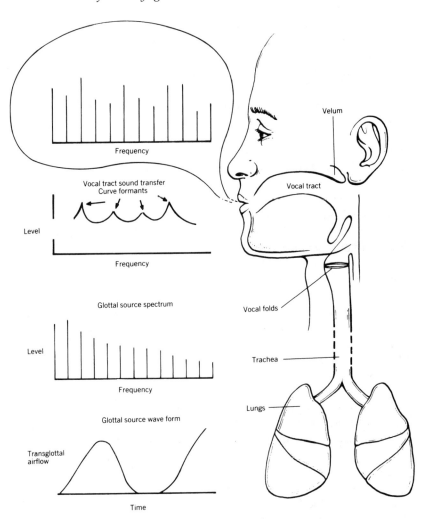

FIG 2-7. Determinants of the spectrum of a vowel (oral-output signal). (From Sataloff R, *Professional Voice: The Science and Art of Clinical Care.* 2nd ed. San Diego: Singular Publishing Group; 1997:168, with permission.)

the cricothyroid muscle makes the thyroid cartilage pivot, increasing the distance between the thyroid and arytenoid cartilages and consequently stretching the vocal folds. This increases the surface area exposed to subglottal pressure and makes the air pressure more effective in opening the vocal folds. In addition, the elastic fibers of the vocal folds are stretched, making them more efficient at snapping back together. Hence, the cycles shorten, repeat more frequently, and the fundamental frequency and pitch rise. Other muscles, including the thyroarytenoid, also contribute. Raising the pressure of the air stream also tends to increase fundamental frequency, a phenomenon for which singers must compensate. Otherwise, their pitch would go up whenever they tried to sing more loudly.

Vocal intensity, which corresponds to loudness, depends on the degree to which the glottal wave excites the air in the vocal tract. Raising the air pressure creates greater amplitude of vocal fold vibration and, consequently, increased vocal intensity. However, it is not the vibrating vocal fold but rather the sudden cessation of airflow that is responsible for establishing acoustic vibration in the vocal tract and controlling intensity. This is similar to the mechanism of acoustic vibration from hand clapping. In the larynx, the sharper the flow cutoff, the more intense the sounds. In fact, great vocal intensity is marked primarily by a steeper closing phase of the glottal wave, achieved by both higher air pressure and biomechanical vocal fold changes that increase glottal resistance to airflow. Assessing an individual's ability to optimize adjustments of air pressure and glottal resistance may be helpful in identifying and correcting voice dysfunction. If high subglottic pressure is combined with high adductory vocal fold force, glottal airflow and the amplitude of the voice source fundamental frequency are low. This is called *pressed phonation* and can be measured clinically through flow glottography. Flow glottography employs inverse filtering of the supraglottic contribution to voice to generate a wave that describes voice source signal characteristics. Flow glottogram wave amplitude indicates the type of phonation being used, and the slope (closing rate) provides information about the sound pressure level or loudness. If adductory forces are so weak that the vocal folds do not make contact, the glottis becomes inefficient and the voice source fundamental is also low. This is known as *breathy phonation*. *Flow phonation* is characterized by lower subglottic pressure and lower adductory force. These conditions increase the dominance of the fundamental frequency of the voice source. Sundberg has shown that the amplitude of the fundamental frequency can be increased by 15 dB or more when changing from pressed phonation to flow phonation. If a patient habitually uses pressed phonation, considerable effort will be required to achieve loud voicing. The muscle patterns and force recruitment often used to compensate for this laryngeal inefficiency may cause vocal damage.

REFERENCES

1. Sundberg J. *The Science of the Singing Voice.* DeKalb, Ill: Northern Illinois University Press; 1987.

2. Scherer RS. Physiology of phonation: a review of basic mechanics. In: Ford CN, Bless DM, eds. *Phonosurgery.* New York, NY: Raven Press; 1991:77–93.
3. Sataloff RT. Clinical anatomy and physiology of the voice. In: Sataloff RT, *Professional Voice: The Science and Art of Clinical Care.* 2nd ed. San Diego, Calif: Singular Publishing Group; 1997:93–190.
4. Garrett JD, Larson CR. Neurology of the laryngeal cisson. In: Ford CN, Bless DM, eds. *Phonosurgery.* New York, NY: Raven Press; 1991:43–76.
5. Hirano M. Phonosurgery. Basic and clinical investigations. *Otologia (Fukuoka).* 1975; 21:239–442.

CHAPTER 3

Anatomy and Physiology of the Esophagus and Its Sphincters

ANATOMY

The human esophagus is a muscular tube whose major function is transport of food from the mouth to the stomach. It is bounded by a tonically contracted circular muscle sphincter at each end. The median length of the esophageal body between the two sphincters is 22 cm in adult females and 24 cm in males. Individual variations in length are normally distributed in both genders[1] (Fig 3-1). The upper esophageal sphincter (UES) consists primarily of striated muscle of the cricopharyngeus muscle, but is enhanced by the inferior pharyngeal constrictors and the circular muscles of the upper esophagus. The anterior attachment of the cricopharyngeus to the cricoid cartilage of the larynx results in the strongest contractile force of this sphincter occurring in the anterior-posterior direction, producing a slitlike configuration with the widest portion facing laterally.[2] The UES, like the striated musculature of the tongue, pharynx, and upper portion of the esophagus, is innervated like skeletal muscle, receiving motor input directly from the brain stem (nucleus ambiguus) to the motor end-plates in the muscle. Chronic tone is maintained by continuous stimulation, which is temporarily inhibited during a swallow.

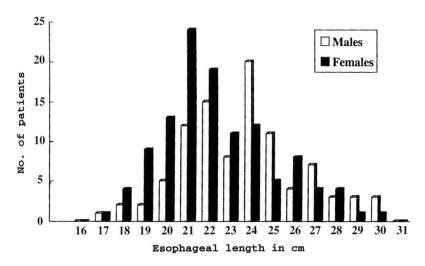

FIG 3-1. Distribution of esophageal length in 212 patients and normal volunteers. Males are shown in white, females in black. Approximation to a normal distribution is verified by similar means and mediums (males: mean = 23.6 cm, median = 24.0 cm; females: mean = 22.4 cm, median = 22.0 cm).

The lower esophageal sphincter (LES), like most of the gastrointestinal (GI) tract, consists entirely of smooth muscle. This sphincter is much more rounded in its closure, yet still demonstrates some degree of radial asymmetry, having higher pressures in the posterolateral direction.[3] Innervation of the LES originates from the dorsal motor nucleus of the brain stem and the efferent fibers are carried through the vagus nerve and synapse in the myenteric plexus in the region of the LES.

The muscular wall of the esophagus is composed of an inner circular and an outer longitudinal layer, with no serosa overlying the muscle layers. The UES and the upper portion of the tubular esophagus are primarily striated muscle. Recent studies have indicated that the transition from predominately striated to predominately smooth muscle occurs in the upper 4 to 5 cm of the human esophagus, although it is quite variable in different subjects and in the different muscle layers. Consistently, greater than the distal half of the human esophagus is entirely smooth muscle.[4] Like the LES, the smooth muscle portion of the tubular esophagus is innervated primarily via the vagus nerve from neurons arising in the dorsal motor nucleus connecting to the myenteric plexus.

PHYSIOLOGY

Swallowing, or deglutition, has 3 stages: the oral (voluntary) stage, the pharyngeal (involuntary) stage, and the esophageal stage. These 3 closely coordinated and merged processes are regulated through the swallowing center in the medulla.[5]

Oral Stage

This preparatory stage includes mechanical disruption of the food and mixing with salivary bicarbonate and enzymes (amylase, lipase). It is an essential process by which the swallowing mechanism is primed. Ingested food is voluntarily moved posteriorly by pistonlike movements of the tongue muscles, forcing the food bolus toward the pharynx and pushing it backward and upward against the palate. Once the food has been delivered to the pharynx, the process becomes involuntary. The oral, preparatory stage obviously requires proper functioning of the striated muscles of the tongue and pharynx and is the stage of swallowing that is likely to be abnormal in patients with neurologic or skeletal muscle disease. Appropriate mentation is also necessary.

Pharyngeal Stage

During this stage of swallowing, the food is passed from the pharynx, across the UES, and into the proximal esophagus. This involuntary process requires the finely tuned coordinated sequences of contraction and relaxation, resulting in *transfer* of the ingested material, while protecting the airway. The presence of food in the pharynx stimulates sensory receptors, which send impulses to the swallowing center in the brain stem. The central nervous system (CNS) then initiates a series of involuntary responses that include the following:

1. The soft palate is pulled upward and *closes the posterior nares.*
2. The palatopharyngeal folds are pulled medially, limiting the opening through the pharynx.
3. The vocal folds are closed and the epiglottis swings backward and down *to close the larynx.*
4. The larynx is pulled upward and forward by the muscles attached to the hyoid bone, stretching the opening of the esophagus and UES.
5. The *UES relaxes. Active relaxation* of the usually tonic cricopharyngeus is essential to permit the passive opening of the UES created by the movement of the larynx.
6. Peristaltic contraction of the constrictor muscles of the pharynx produces the force that propels food into the esophagus.

This sequence is a coordinated mechanism that includes impulses carried by 5 cranial nerves. Sensory information to the swallowing center is carried along cranial nerves V, VII, IX, and X. The motor responses from the swallowing center are carried along cranial nerves V, VII, IX, X, and XII and also the ansa cervicalis (C-1 and C-2). This intricate process takes just over 1 second from start to finish and requires coordination of pharyngeal contraction and UES relaxation (Fig 3-2). The UES is only open for approximately 500 milliseconds.

Esophageal Stage

The main function of the esophagus is to *transport* ingested material from the mouth to the stomach. This active process requires contraction of both longitudinal and circular muscles of the tubular esophagus and coordinated relaxation of the sphincters. At the onset of swallowing, the longitudinal muscle contracts and shortens the esophagus to provide a structural base for the circular muscle contraction that forms the peristaltic wave. The sequential contraction of esophageal circular smooth muscle from proximal to distal generates the peristaltic clearing wave. The neuromuscular control of this activity will be described below. As opposed to other GI tract smooth muscle, the esophageal smooth muscle has a unique electrical activity pattern, showing only spiked potentials without underlying slow waves. Circular muscle contractions can be characterized into 3 distinct patterns.

1. *Primary peristalsis.* This is the usual form of contraction wave of circular muscle that progresses down the esophagus and is initiated by the central mechanisms that follow the voluntary act of swallowing. It follows sequentially the pressure generated in the pharynx and requires approximately 8 to 10 seconds to reach the distal esophagus. The LES relaxes at the onset of the swallow and remains relaxed until it contracts as a continuation of the progressive peristaltic wave. These pressure relationships are shown in Fig 3-3.
2. *Secondary peristalsis.* This represents a peristaltic contraction of the circular esophageal muscle, which begins without central stimulation. This is to say, it originates in the esophagus as a result of distention and will usually continue until the esophagus is empty. Some food, particularly solid material, requires more than the single primary peristaltic wave for eventual clearance. This is accomplished by the secondary peristaltic waves. Thus, secondary peristalsis is the mechanism for clearing both ingested material and also material that is refluxed from the stomach. Experimentally, secondary peristalsis can be demonstrated by inflating a balloon in the mid- to upper esophagus.

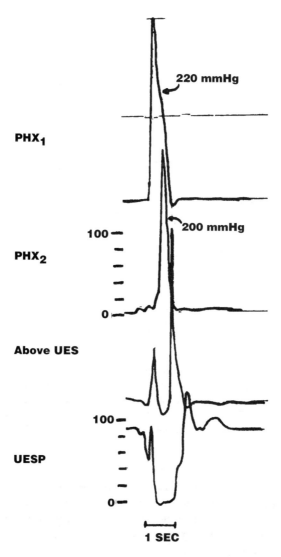

FIG 3-2. Motility tracing showing the coordinated sequence of contraction of the human pharynx and relaxation of the UES. The 4 recording sites are spaced at 3-cm intervals, with the lowest in the UES high pressure zone (UESP), the second from bottom located just proximal to the UES, and the next 2 sites at 3-cm (PHX_2) and 6-cm (PHX_1) distances proximally. The sequential contraction in the pharynx is noted in the 2 proximal recording sites. Movement of the UES orad followed by UES relaxation and subsequent descent of the UES during the swallow generates the "M" configuration shown at the third recording site. The apparently longer UES "relaxation" seen in the distal sensor is an artifact produced by the movement of the sphincter orad away from the transducer during swallowing. The actual time of UES relaxation is approximately 0.5 seconds as shown in the recording located second from the bottom.

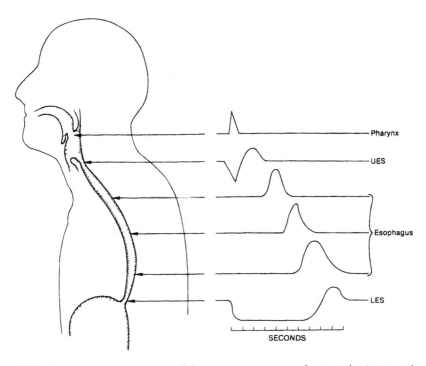

FIG 3-3. Schematic presentation of the pressure sequence of a normal primary peristaltic wave. Note the pressure complex that begins in the pharynx and progressively closes off the UES, then moves sequentially down the esophageal body and closes the LES. Also note that LES relaxation begins with the onset of the swallow and remains relaxed until the peristaltic wave reaches the distal esophagus (8-10 seconds).

3. *Tertiary contractions.* This contraction pattern is identified primarily during barium x-ray studies of the esophagus. It represents a non-peristaltic series of contraction waves that appear as localized segmented indentations in the barium column. It has no known physiologic function.

One of the interesting phenomena seen in the human esophagus occurs during the process of rapid sequential swallowing (10 seconds or less between successive voluntary swallows). This process results in inhibition of peristalsis, so-called "deglutitive inhibition." Peristalsis will be suspended during the continuation of a series of rapid swallows and a large "clearing wave" will occur at the completion of the swallows (Fig 3-4). This phenomenon occurs because of the inhibitory neural discharge that arises from the central swallowing center during

Anatomy and Physiology of the Esophagus and Its Sphincters

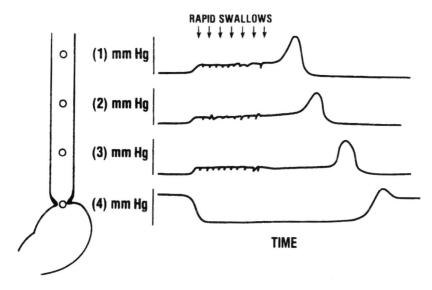

FIG 3-4. Demonstration of the phenomenon of deglutitive inhibition of the peristaltic sequence by rapid swallows separated by approximately 5-second intervals. The LES remains relaxed throughout the sequence as the esophageal body is inhibited from a peristaltic response until the termination of the swallows. At this point the peristaltic clearing wave occurs.

swallowing, and also because the esophageal musculature shows a refractoriness, demonstrated to persist for up to 10 seconds.[6]

Importance of the Sphincters

The esophagus is located in the thorax and has negative pressure relative to pressures in the pharynx proximally and the stomach distally. Therefore, the sphincters must maintain constant closure to prevent abnormal movement of air or food into the esophagus. In the absence of a tonically contracted UES, air will flow freely into the esophagus during inspiration. In the presence of a weak LES, gastric contents are not inhibited from refluxing into the distal esophagus, particularly in the recumbent position. Pressure relationships in and around the esophagus and its sphincters are shown in Fig 3-5.

Upper Esophageal Sphincter

The UES maintains a constant closure with strongest forces directed in the anterior-posterior orientation as a result of the sling-shaped

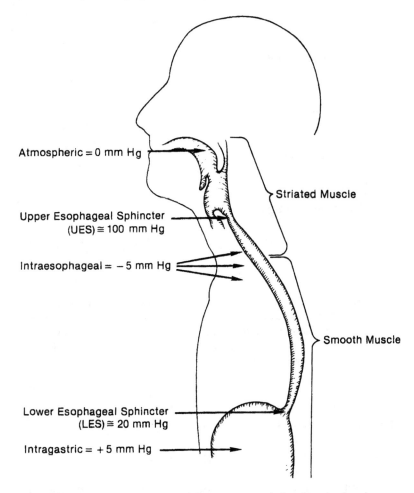

FIG 3-5. Schematic representation of the pressure relationships in the pharynx, esophagus, esophageal sphincters, and stomach. Note the negative intraesophageal pressure relative to both pharyngeal (atmospheric) pressure and intragastric pressure. Thus, the importance of the sphincters in prevention of abnormal movement of fluids and air is emphasized.

attachment of the cricopharyngeus to the cricoid cartilage. Normal pressures in the UES are approximately 100 mm Hg in the anterior-posterior direction and approximately 50 mm Hg laterally.[2]

Lower Esophageal Sphincter

The tonically contracted LES normally maintains a closing pressure 10 to 45 mm Hg greater than the intragastric pressure below. By convention, LES pressure is measured as a gradient in mm Hg higher than intragastric pressure, which is used as a zero reference. At the time of swallowing, the LES relaxes promptly in response to the initial neural discharge from the swallowing center and stays relaxed until the peristaltic wave reaches the end of the esophagus and produces sphincter closure. During relaxation, the pressure measured within the sphincter falls approximately to the level of gastric pressure; this is by definition a "complete" relaxation. Although there has been much controversy over the years, it is now generally accepted that the LES does *not* have to be located within the diaphragmatic crus to maintain a constant closing pressure. Thus, the presence of a sliding hiatal hernia is not necessarily detrimental to the physiologic function of this sphincter.

The LES maintains two important physiologic functions; the first is its role in prevention of gastroesophageal reflux and the second is its ability to relax with swallowing to allow movement of ingested material into the stomach. The mechanism by which the circular smooth muscle of the LES maintains tonic closure has been a subject of considerable investigation over many years. At present, this is felt to be predominantly the result of intrinsic muscle activity, since investigations in animals have demonstrated that resting LES tone persists even after the destruction of all neural input by the neurotoxin tetrodotoxin.[7] In addition, truncal vagotomy does not affect resting LES pressure in humans. Calcium channel-blocking agents, which exert their effect directly on the circular smooth muscle, will produce decreases in LES pressures in animals and humans.[8,9] There also appears to be some cholinergic tone present in many animal species and in humans, as atropine or injection of botulinum toxin will produce marked decreases in resting LES pressure.[10,11]

The mechanism of relaxation of the LES in response to a swallow has also been a subject of considerable investigation and controversy. The precise neurotransmitter responsible for this response is not definitely known. It is clear that it is not a classic cholinergic or adrenergic agent because specific pharmacologic blockade of these mechanisms does not inhibit LES relaxation. This is a neural event, however, because it can be reproduced in animals by stimulation of the vagus nerve and relaxation is inhibited by tetrodotoxin.[12] These relationships are summarized in Fig 3-6. Recent studies indicate that the neurotransmitter might be a combination of vasoactive intestinal polypeptide (VIP) and nitric oxide.[12,13]

LES resting pressure is dynamic and demonstrates frequent changes. Pressures measured over long periods of time indicate that LES pressure will vary considerably, even from minute to minute. Much of this is due to the effect of a variety of factors that modulate

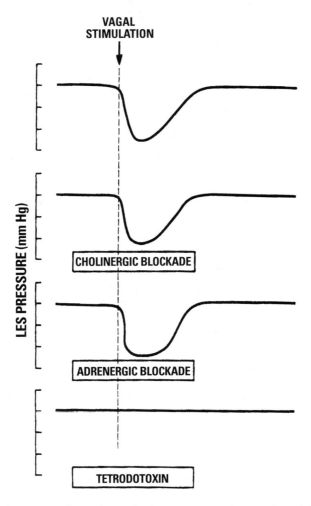

FIG 3-6. Summation of experiments in the opossum on the neural regulation of LES relaxation. Electrical stimulation of the vagus nerve produces relaxation, which is not inhibited by blocking either cholinergic or adrenergic pathways. However, the neural response is inhibited by the neurotoxin tetrodotoxin.

pressure. These include foods ingested during meals and other events such as cigarette smoking and gastric distention. The normal LES will respond to transient increases in intra-abdominal pressure by raising its resting pressure to a greater degree than the pressure increases in

Anatomy and Physiology of the Esophagus and Its Sphincters

the abdomen below. This normal protective mechanism guards against gastroesophageal reflux. In addition, many hormones and other peptide substances produced in the GI tract and in other areas of the body have been shown to affect LES pressure. These are summarized in Table 3-1. Many of these likely represent pharmacologic responses that have been shown to occur after intravenous injections or infusions of these substances in man or animals. Whether they represent truly physiologic actions has not been clarified in most cases. The strongest candidates for physiologic hormonal control of the LES are cholecystokinin, which helps explain the decreases in LES pressures seen after fat ingestion, and progesterone, which explains the decreases in LES pressure that occur during pregnancy. Finally, various neurotransmitters and pharmacologic agents have been shown to affect LES pressure. These are summarized in Table 3-2. The modulation of LES resting pressure is a complex mechanism that involves the interaction of the LES smooth muscle, neural control, and humeral factors.[14]

Controls of Esophageal Peristalsis

As noted above, esophageal peristalsis is controlled via afferent and efferent neural connections through the swallowing center in the medulla. This central mechanism regulates the involuntary sequence of muscular events that occurs during swallowing and simultaneously inhibits the respiratory center in the medulla so that respiration is stopped during the pharyngeal stage of swallowing.

The direct innervation to the striated muscle area of the pharynx and upper esophagus is carried via fibers from the brain stem (nucleus ambiguus) through the vagus nerve. The innervation to the smooth muscle of the distal esophagus and LES arises from the dorsal motor nucleus of the vagus and is carried through cholinergic visceral motor

TABLE 3-1. *Effects of Peptides and Hormones on LES Pressure*

Increases LES	Decreases LES
Gastrin	Secretin
Motilin	Cholecystokinin
Substance P	Glucagon
Pancreatic polypeptide	Gastric inhibitory polypeptide (GIP)
Bombesin	Vasoactive intestinal polypeptide (VIP)
Leu-enkephalin	Peptide histidine isoleucine
Pitressin	Progesterone
Angiotensin	

TABLE 3-2. Effects of Neurotransmitters and Pharmacologic Agents on LES Pressure

Increases LES	Decreases LES
Cholinergic (bethanechol)	Nitric oxide
(x-Adrenergic)	Dopamine
Metoclopramide	P-Adrenergic
Cisapride	Atropine
	Nitrates
	Calcium-channel blockers
	Morphine
	Valium
	Theophylline

nerves to ganglia in the myenteric plexus (Auerbach). Noncholinergic, nonadrenergic inhibitory nerves are also carried within the vagus.

The myenteric plexus in the esophageal portion of the enteric nervous system (the "brain in the gut") receives efferent impulses from the CNS and sensory afferents from the esophagus. Thus, impulses travel in two directions through this modulating area, which interconnects and regulates signals that result in normal peristalsis in the smooth muscle esophagus. One manifestation of the afferent control is the regulation of peristaltic squeezing pressures, to some degree, by the size of the ingested bolus. In addition, dry swallows often fail to provide adequate stimulation for the production of complete esophageal peristaltic pressures. The importance of the myenteric plexus as the primary regulatory mechanism of esophageal peristalsis in the smooth muscle portion is shown by observations that bilateral cervical vagotomy in animals does not abolish peristalsis in this area.

Interesting results have been obtained from in vitro studies of esophageal smooth-muscle preparations.[15] Using muscle from the opossum esophagus, it has been shown that the longitudinal smooth muscle demonstrates a sustained contraction during electrical field stimulation; this is called the "duration response." This response is neural and cholinergic since it can be blocked with both atropine and tetrodotoxin. The circular smooth muscle of the opossum esophagus shows a quite different response. With the onset of electrical stimulation there is a brief, small contraction at the beginning of the stimulus, known as the "on-response." This response is quite variable and has no known physiologic role. The on-response is followed by a much larger contraction that occurs after the termination of the stimulus, known as the "off-response." This response is also neural in origin, but is not cholinergic, since it is blocked only by tetrodotoxin and not atropine. Muscle strips taken from different segments of the smooth muscle portion of the esophageal body show progressively longer intervals for the off-response contraction following stimulation as one moves distally in the esophagus. This phenomenon has been called the "latency gradient." These concepts are shown in Fig 3-7.

It has been proposed that these in vitro experiments from the opossum esophagus may help to explain some of the mechanisms of the development of normal peristalsis in the human smooth-muscle esophagus. With the initial swallowing event, an inhibitory neural discharge is sent to the circular smooth muscle of the entire esophagus. The LES relaxes from its resting tonic state. The remainder of the esophageal smooth muscle is already relaxed and shows no measurable change. Rebound contraction occurs following the end of the brief stimulus (the off-response). The latency of the gradient for this off-response, progressing distally down the esophagus, produces the peristaltic contraction wave. Although this concept does not entirely explain all of the phenomena that have been observed in human peristaltic activity, these in vitro observations are consistent with many aspects of normal human physiology. One example is the deglutitive inhibition referred to above. With repetitive swallowing at frequent

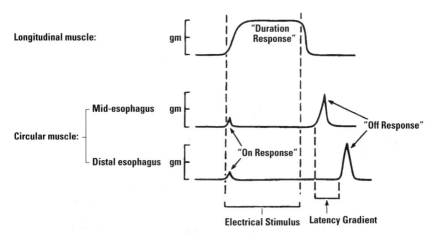

FIG 3-7. Summary of the in vitro esophageal smooth-muscle responses shown in experiments in the opossum. During stimulation the longitudinal esophageal muscle contracts throughout the stimulus; this is known as the duration response. The circular muscle shows a brief positive impulse at the beginning of stimulation; this is known as the on-response. This is followed by a much greater contraction following termination of the stimulus; this is known as the off-response. Delay in the latter response, progressing daily in the esophagus, produces the so-called latency gradient (gm = contraction force in grams).

intervals, the successive inhibitory neural impulses from the swallowing center prevent the contractions of the smooth-muscle portion of the esophagus until the last swallow occurs. The off-response and the latency gradient then allow the single peristaltic clearing wave that usually follows.

REFERENCES

1. Li Q, Castell JA, Castell DO. Manometric determination of esophageal length. *Am J Gastroenterol*. 1994; 89:722–725.
2. Gerhardt DC, Shuck TL, Bordeaux RA, et al. Human upper esophageal sphincter. *Gastroenterology*. 1978;75:268–274.
3. Winans CS. Manometric asymmetry of the lower esophageal high pressure zone. *Am J Dig Dis*. 1977;22:348–354.
4. Meyer GW, Austin RM, Brady CE, et al. Muscle anatomy of the human esophagus. *J Clin Gastroenterol*. 1986;8:131–137.
5. Weisbrodt NW. Neuromuscular organization of esophageal and pharyngeal motility. *Arch Intern Med*. 1967;136:524–531.
6. Meyer GW, Gerhardt DC, Castell DO. Human esophageal response to rapid swallowing: muscle refractory period or neural inhibition? *Am J Physiol*. 1981;241:Gl29–Gl36.
7. Goyal RK, Rattan S. Genesis of basal sphincter pressure: effect of tetrodotoxin on the lower esophageal sphincter in opossum in vivo. *Gastroenterology*. 1976;71:62–67.
8. Richter JE, Sinar DR, Cordova CM, et al. Verapamil—a potent inhibitor of esophageal function in baboons. *Gastroenterology*. 1982;82:882–886.
9. Richter JE, Spurling TJ, Cordova CM, et al. Effects of oral calcium blocker, diltiazem, on esophageal contractions. *Dig Dis Sci*. 1984;29:649–656.
10. Dodds WJ, Dent J, Hogan WJ, et al. Effect of atropine on esophageal motor function in humans. *Am J Physiol*. 1981;240:G290–G296.
11. Pasricha PJ, Ravich WJ, Kalloo AN. Effects of intragastric botulinum toxin on the lower esophageal sphincter in piglets. *Gastroenterology*. 1993; 105:1045–1049.
12. Goyal RK, Rattan S, Said SI. VIP as a possible neurotransmitter of non-cholinergic non-adrenergic inhibitory neurons. *Nature*. 1980;288:370–380.
13. Sanders KM, Ward SM. Nitric oxide as a mediator of nonadrenergic non-cholinergic neurotransmission. *Am J Physiol*. 1992;262:G379–G392.
14. Castell DO. The lower esophageal sphincter: physiologic and clinical aspects. *Ann Intern Med*. 1975;83:390–401.
15. Christensen J, Lund GF. Esophageal responses to distention and electrical stimulation. *J Clin Invest*. 1969;48:408–419.

CHAPTER 4

Gastroesophageal Reflux Disease: An Overview of Clinical Presentation and Epidemiology

Gastroesophageal reflux disease (GERD) is a spectrum of disease best defined as symptoms and/or signs of esophageal or adjacent organ injury, secondary to the reflux of gastric contents into the esophagus or beyond into the oral cavity or airways. GERD is a common disorder seen in all clinical practice and presents with a multitude of symptoms. Injury is defined based on symptoms or organ damage resulting in esophagitis, inflammation of the larynx and oropharynx, or acute and/or chronic pulmonary injury. This chapter presents an overview of GERD including typical, atypical, and extra-esophageal presentations.

TYPICAL SYMPTOMS

The typical or classic symptoms are heartburn, defined as substernal burning occurring shortly after meals or on bending over and relieved with antacids and regurgitation (the spontaneous return of gastric contents into the esophagus or mouth). When present together, heartburn and regurgitation establish the diagnosis with greater than 90% certainty. Heartburn is seen daily in 7% to 10% of the population in the United States and at least monthly in about 40% to 50%.[1-3] Over 20 million people in the U.S. have heartburn at least twice a week and use antacids or other over-the-counter antireflux products on a regular basis. Regurgitation is experienced weekly by about 6% of the population according to one recent study.[2] In the same study, either heartburn or regurgitation was present weekly in 20% of patients surveyed and monthly in 59%. The prevalence of heartburn appears to decrease slightly with increasing age.

Classic heartburn is described by the patient as a burning sensation under the breast bone with radiation upward toward the throat or mouth. Heartburn occurs 1 to 2 hours after meals, with heavy lifting, or on bending over. Big meals, spicy foods, citrus products, such as a grapefruit and orange juice, and meals high in fat are more likely to produce symptoms. Colas, coffee, teas, and even beer may have acidic pH and cause symptoms when ingested. Meals eaten late in the evening, close to bedtime, or taken with alcohol make patients more prone to nighttime symptoms. Patients will often describe their symptoms as relieved with an over-the-counter antacid preparation, H_2-receptor antagonist, or even drinking water. Heartburn may be exacerbated by many foods, drugs or by exercise (Table 4-1).

While heartburn is often associated with the presence of regurgitation, the spontaneous appearance of an acid or bitter taste in the chest or mouth, these are not synonymous symptoms. Heartburn (pyrosis) should not be confused with dyspepsia, a more vague epigastric distress usually localized in the upper abdominal or lower substernal area and associated with nausea, bloating, or fullness after meals. Although dyspepsia may be a symptom of GERD, it is neither as sensitive nor as specific as heartburn. The generic use of acid indigestion to encompass all symptoms related to GERD is inappropriate; these symptoms must be distinguished for accurate diagnosis and therapy. Waterbrash, the sudden filling of the mouth with a clear, salty fluid, should not be confused with heartburn. This symptom reflects the increase in salivary secretion seen as a reflex response to reflux or regurgitation of gastric acid into a inflamed distal esophagus.

Heartburn is a highly specific symptom for GERD; its presence is almost always diagnostic. One major exception can occur; a heartburn-like symptom, suspected to be due to esophageal stasis from outflow obstruction, is often described in patients with achalasia. It is felt that fermentation of undigested food in the esophagus coupled with inflammation may create a heartburnlike sensation in the absence of true

TABLE 4-1. *Factors Causing Exacerbation of Heartburn*

Decreases LES Pressure	Mucosal Irritant
Food	Food and drinks
Fats	Citrus products
Chocolate	Tomato products
Onions	Spicy foods
Carminatives	Coffee, colas, tea, beer
Coffee	Medications
Alcohol	Aspirin
Smoking	NSAIDs
Medications	Tetracycline
Progesterone	Quinidine
Theophylline	Potassium tablets
Anticholinergic agents	Iron salts
b-Adrenergic agonists	Alendronate
a-Adrenergic antagonists	Zidovudine
Diazepam	
Meperidine	
Nitrates	
Calcium channel blockers	

LES = lower esophageal sphincter; NSAIDs = nonsteroidal anti-inflammatory drugs.

GERD. With this major exception, if heartburn is the only presenting esophageal symptom, it is likely due to GERD.

Despite the sensitivity and specificity of these 2 symptoms for the diagnosis of GERD, neither the *presence* of heartburn and/or regurgitation nor the *frequency* of these symptoms is predictive of the degree of endoscopic damage to the distal esophagus. The frequency of heartburn usually does not correlate with the severity of GERD, although nocturnal heartburn suggests the possibility of erosive esophagitis. Only 50% to 60% of patients presenting to a physician with heartburn will have erosive esophagitis seen on a diagnostic endoscopic examination; the remainder will be diagnosed as having nonerosive GERD.[4] Severe disease including Barrett's esophagus and peptic strictures may present with infrequent or absent complaints of heartburn, while many patients with daily heartburn will have no endoscopic abnormalities.

Most patients with esophagitis will not progress beyond the endoscopic stage seen at initial endoscopy. In a series of 701 patients followed for up to 29 years, only 23% progressed to a more serious grade of esophagitis.[5] The patient with reflux symptoms and *no* esophagitis (nonerosive GERD) has even less likelihood of progression, with less than 15% of patients progressing to a higher grade over 6 months.[6]

Regurgitation, the effortless return of gastric contents into the esophagus or the mouth, is often associated with heartburn and GERD. When the two symptoms are present together the diagnosis of GERD is highly likely. Regurgitation without heartburn should raise suspicion of Barrett's esophagus (in which acid sensitivity is reduced), achalasia, or other esophageal obstruction. Regurgitation may also be seen as a more prominent symptom in extra-esophageal manifestations of GERD, particularly pulmonary related symptoms; and it may be an important prognostic factor in predicting outcome of therapy.[7,8] Regurgitation is often confused by patients as vomiting. The effortless return of food or fluid in the absence of nausea is an important distinction between these 2 symptoms. Symptoms associated with GERD are outlined in Table 4-2.

EXTRA-ESOPHAGEAL (ATYPICAL) SYMPTOMS

A number of so-called atypical or extra-esophageal symptoms have been associated with GERD, including unexplained subsernal chest pain without evidence of coronary artery disease (noncardiac chest pain), asthma, bronchitis, chronic cough, recurrent pneumonia, hoarseness, chronic posterior laryngitis, globus sensation, otalgia, apthous ulcers, hiccups, and erosion of dental enamel. In contrast to heartburn and regurgitation, the prevalence of these atypical or extra-esophageal symptoms and their frequency in the general population has not been systematically studied until recently. In a large population-based survey of Caucasians in Olmstead County, Minnesota,[2] designed to assess the prevalence of GERD in the general population, unexplained chest pain was seen in 23% of the population yearly and in 4% at least weekly. The frequency of unexplained chest pain surprisingly decreased with age. Forty percent had symptoms for more than 5 years

TABLE 4-2. *Symptoms Associated with Gastroesophageal Reflux*

Esophageal	Extra-esophageal
Heartburn	Hoarseness
Regurgitation	Chronic cough
Dysphagia	Laryngitis or laryngospasm
Odynophagia (rare)	Asthma or respiratory disease
Waterbrash	Vocal fold granulomas
Chest pain	Loss of dental enamel
	Otalgia
	Nausea

and 5% reported severe symptoms. Asthma was reported in approximately 9%, bronchitis in approximately 20%, and chronic hoarseness in 15% of patients who had typical GERD symptoms.

The association of these atypical symptoms with heartburn and regurgitation is controversial. In the Minnesota study,[2] patients with heartburn and regurgitation had one or more atypical symptoms about 80% of the time. Atypical symptoms were more common in patients with frequent GERD compared to patients with no GERD symptoms. The only exception was asthma. Heartburn or regurgitation was reported in more than 80% of the patients with unexplained chest pain and in 60% with globus sensation. Approximately 60% of patients with asthma, bronchitis, hoarseness, and pneumonia had heartburn or regurgitation. The presence of heartburn is not predictive of otolaryngologic symptoms. However, in a recent case control study from the Veterans Administration, patients with a discharge diagnosis of erosive esophagitis had twice the prevalence of an associated otolaryngologic symptom as control patients without esophagitis.[9] Observations in patients presenting with atypical GERD are that frequent heartburn and regurgitation are uncommon complaints; however, the absence of these typical symptoms should not preclude making a diagnosis. Prospective studies using endoscopy and ambulatory pH monitoring find GERD in as many as 75% of patients with chronic hoarseness,[10] between 70% and 80% of asthmatics,[11,12] and 20% of patients with chronic cough.[13] Approximately 45% of patients with unexplained chest pain can be shown to have GERD.[14] Esophagitis in this population is less common, being seen in less than 10%.[15] Endoscopic esophagitis is seen in 30% to 40% of patients with asthma[16,17] and about 20% of patients with reflux laryngitis. Distinguishing between cardiac and noncardiac chest pain due to GERD is difficult, and they may coexist in the same patient. All of the features of cardiac angina—tight, gripping viselike pain radiating to the neck, shoulder, or left arm and associated with exertion—may be seen with GERD. Long episodes of pain (greater than 1 hour), pain relieved by eating or pain awakening from sleep are more likely esophageal. Antacids or H_2-blockers may relieve chest pain later proven to be associated with coronary artery disease. It is therefore crucial to rule out cardiac disease before presuming GERD as the cause of chest pain.

Seventy to 80% of patients with asthma will have associated GERD. Whether this is cause and effect or coincident presence of 2 diseases is not clear. A careful history will reveal heartburn or regurgitation in only 50%. Onset of asthma late in life, the absence of a seasonal or allergic component, and onset after a big meal or alcohol suggest GERD-related asthma. Reflux is the third most common cause of chronic cough, after postnasal drip and bronchitis. In the patient with cough, a normal chest X ray, and no postnasal drip, GERD should be considered as the most likely diagnosis.

Hoarseness is the most common otolaryngologic symptom of GERD. Most studies suggest that heartburn is present in only about 50%. In our experience a careful history will discover heartburn to be present in about 75%.[21] Other associated symptoms include halitosis, throat clearing, dry cough, coated tongue, globus sensation, tickle in the throat, chronic sore throat, postnasal drip, and others discussed in Chapter 5. Difficulty in warming up the voice in the professional singer, early voice fatigue, and intermittent laryngitis are associated symptoms. Erosion of dental enamel may be due to GERD; however, its frequency is not known.

COMPLICATIONS OF GERD

GERD may present with severe complications, including peptic stricture, ulceration, iron deficiency anemia, or most importantly Barrett's esophagus, the change from normal squamous epithelial lining to a metaplastic intestinal type epithelium with typical special staining characteristics—a premalignant condition. Estimates are that 2% to 10% of patients with GERD will have strictures [18] and 10% to 15% will have Barrett's esophagus.[4,19] Dysphagia, odynophagia (painful swallowing), and bleeding suggest complicated GERD. Slowly progressive dysphagia, particularly for solids, suggests peptic strictures. Liquid and solid dysphagia suggests a GERD-related motility disorder secondary to erosive esophagitis, Barrett's esophagus, or scleroderma. GERD-related motility disorders are seen in increased frequency in patients with otolaryngologic GERD,[20] even though dysphagia is not usually a presenting symptom. Motility abnormalities have important complications for the patient considering surgery (see Chapter 7). Odynophagia is rare in reflux. Its presence suggests ulceration or inflammation and it is seen most frequently in infectious or pill-induced esophagitis. Occasionally esophagitis may present with occult, upper GI bleeding or iron deficiency anemia.[18] The frequency of these complications in patients with reflux laryngitis is not known.

GERD IS A CHRONIC DISEASE

There is ample evidence that patients with reflux esophagitis will have endoscopic and symptomatic relapse up to 80% of the time if therapy is discontinued or drug dosage is decreased. Studies of patients with otolaryngologic manifestations of GERD suggest similar findings.

Recurrence of hoarseness was seen within 6 months in one study.[22] The clinical impression is that all GERD is chronic, with individuals expressing this chronicity in different ways. Most patients, especially those with extra-esophageal disease, will require long-term therapy or surgery to achieve adequate symptom relief.

REFERENCES

1. *A Gallup Survey on Heartburn Across America.* New York, NY: The Gallup Organization Inc; 1968.
2. Locke GR, Talley NJ, Fett SL, Zinsmeister AR, Melton LJ. Prevalence and clinical spectrum of gastroesophageal reflux: a population-based study in Olmstead County, Minnesota. *Gastroenterology.* 1997;112:5–12.
3. Nebel OT, Fornes MF, Castell DO. Symptomatic gastroesophageal reflux: incidence and precipitating factors. *Dig Dis Sci.* 1976;21:953–956.
4. Winters C, Spurling TJ, Chobanian SJ, et al. Barrett's esophagus: a prevalent, occult complication of gastroesophageal reflux disease. *Gastroenterology.* 1987;92:118–123.
5. Ollyo JB, Monnier P, Fontollier C, et al. The natural history, prevalence and incidence of reflux esophagitis. *Gullet.* 1993;3(suppl):3–10.
6. Pace F, Santalucia F, Bianchi Porro G. Natural history of gastroesophageal reflux disease without esophagitis. *Gut.* 1991;32:845–848.
7. Schnatz PF, Castell JA, Castell DO. Pulmonary symptoms associated with gastroesophageal reflux: use of ambulatory pH monitoring to diagnose and to direct therapy. *Am J Gastroenterol.* 1996;91:1715–1718.
8. Harding SM, Richter JE, Bradley L, et al. Asthma and gastroesophageal reflux: acid suppression therapy improves asthma outcome. *Am J Med.* 1996;100:395–405.
9. El Serag HB, Sonnenberg A. Comorbid occurrence of laryngeal or pulmonary disease with esophagitis in United States military veterans. *Gastroenterology.* 1997;113:755–760.
10. Koufman JA. The otolaryngologic manifestations of gastroesophageal reflux disease: a clinical investigation of 225 patients using ambulatory pH monitoring and an experimental investigation of the role of acid and pepsin in the development of laryngeal injury. *Laryngoscope.* 1991;101:1–12.
11. Harding SM, Guzzo MR, Richter JE. Prevalence of GERD in asthmatics without reflux symptoms. *Gastroenterology.* 1997;4:A141.
12. Sontag SJ, O'Connell S, Khandelwal S, et al. Most asthmatics have gastroesophageal reflux with or without bronchodilator therapy. *Gastroenterology.* 1990;99:613–618.
13. Irwin RS, French CL, Curley FJ, Zawacki JK, Bennett FM. Chronic cough due to gastroesophageal reflux. Clinical, diagnostic and pathogenic aspects. *Chest.* 1993;194:1511–1517.
14. Hewson EG, Sinclair JW, Dalton CB, et al. 24 hour esophageal pH monitoring: the most useful test for evaluating non-cardiac chest pain. *Am J Med.* 1991;90:576–583.

15. Cherian P, Smith LF, Bardham KD, Thorpe J, Oakley GD, Dawson D. Esophageal tests in the evaluation of non-cardiac chest pain. *Dis Esophagus.* 1995;8:129–133.
16. Larrain A, Carrasco E, Galleguillos F, et al. Medical and surgical treatment of non-allergic asthma associated with gastroesophageal reflux. *Chest.* 1991;99:1330–1336.
17. Sontag SJ, Schnell TG, Miller TQ, et al. Prevalence of esophagitis in asthmatics. *Gut.* 1992;33:872–876.
18. Spechler SJ. Complications of gastroesophageal reflux disease. In: Castell DO, ed. *The Esophagus.* Boston, Mass: Little, Brown and Company; 1992: 543–556.
19. Lieberman D, A Oehlke M, Helfand M, et al. Risk factors for Barrett's esophagus in community based practice. *Am J Gastroenterol.* 1997;92: 1293–1297.
20. Fouad YM, Koury R, Hattlebakk JG, Katz PO, Castell DO. Ineffective esophageal motility (IEM) is more prevalent in reflux patients with respiratory symptoms. *Gastroenterology.* 1998;114:506.
21. Govil Y, Khoury R, Katz PO, et al. Anti-reflux therapy improves symptoms in patients with reflux laryngitis [abstract]. *Gastroenterology.* 1998;114:562.
22. Kamal PL, Hanon D, Kahrilas PJ. Omeprazole for the treatment of posterior laryngitis. *Am J Med.* 1994;96:321.

CHAPTER 5

Reflux Laryngitis and Other Otolaryngologic Manifestations of Laryngopharyngeal Reflux

Although the majority of otolaryngologists have only begun to acknowledge the importance of reflux in causing otolaryngologic disease, many authors have recognized the association for more than 2 decades.[1-25] Otolaryngologists are becoming increasingly diligent about looking for arytenoid erythema and edema, suspecting laryngopharyngeal reflux (LPR) as the underlying problem and treating it as the primary approach to therapy for various reflux-related conditions.

SYMPTOMS

Common symptoms of reflux laryngitis include morning hoarseness, prolonged voice warm-up time (greater than 20-30 minutes), halitosis, excessive phlegm, frequent throat clearing, dry mouth, coated tongue, sensation of a lump in the throat (globus sensation, although recent observations raise questions about this association), throat tickle, dysphagia, regurgitation of gastric contents, chronic sore throat, possibly geographic tongue, nocturnal cough, chronic or recurrent cough, difficulty breathing (especially at night), aspiration, closing off of the airway (laryngospasm), poorly controlled asthma (which causes dysphonia by interfering with the support mechanism), pneumonia, recurrent airway problems in infants, and occasionally dyspepsia (epigastric discomfort) or pyrosis (heartburn). However, dyspepsia and pyrosis are frequently absent. Interestingly, if patients stop reflux treatment after a few months, classic dyspepsia and pyrosis seem to be present commonly when symptoms recur, although this clinically observed phenomenon has not been studied formally. In addition to prolonged vocal warm-up time, professional singers and actors may also complain of voice practice intolerance, manifested by frequent throat clearing and excessive phlegm, especially during the first 10 to 20 minutes of vocal exercises or songs. Hyperfunctional technique during speaking and especially singing is also associated with reflux laryngitis. This is probably due to the vocalist's tendency to guard against aspiration. Voice professionals can be helped somewhat toward overcoming this secondary muscular tension dysphonia through voice therapy with speech-language pathologists, singing voice specialists, and acting voice specialists, but it is difficult to overcome completely until excellent reflux control has been achieved.

PHYSICAL EXAMINATION

Physical examination of patients with throat and voice complaints must be comprehensive. A thorough head and neck examination is always included, with attention to the ears and hearing, nasal patency, the oral cavity and temporomandibular joints, signs of allergy, the larynx, and neck. At least a limited general physical examination is included to look for signs of systemic dysfunction that may present as throat or voice complaints. More comprehensive specialized physical examinations by medical consultants should be sought when indicated.

Laryngoscopic examination typically reveals erythema and edema of the mucosa overlying the arytenoid cartilages, the posterior aspect of the larynx, and often the posterior portion of the true vocal folds. In severe cases, the erythema and edema may be more extensive. Mild, diffuse, nonspecific laryngitis and halitosis are also commonly present. In some patients with LPR severe enough to involve the oral cavity, there is also loss of dental enamel. Hence, transparency of the lower portion of the central incisors may be seen occasionally in reflux patients, although it may be more common in patients with bulimia and those who habitually eat lemons. When the patient has complaints of vocal difficulties, laryngeal examination may also include formal assessment of the speaking and singing voice and strobovideolaryngoscopy for slow motion evaluation of the vibratory margin of the vocal folds. Objective voice analysis quantifies voice quality, pulmonary function, valvular efficiency of the vocal folds, harmonic spectral characteristics, and neuromuscular function, quantified by laryngeal electromyography (EMG). These aspects of the physical examination and tests of voice function are discussed in Chapter 6 and elsewhere, and they will not be reviewed in this chapter.[26]

PATHOPHYSIOLOGY

Laryngopharyngeal reflux can affect anyone, but it appears particularly common and symptomatic in professional voice users, especially singers. This is true for several reasons. First, the technique of singing involves "support," by the forceful compression of the abdominal muscles designed to push the abdominal contents superiorly and pull the sternum down. This action compresses the air in the thorax and generates a force for the stream of expired air, but it also compresses the stomach and works against the lower esophageal sphincter. Singing is an athletic endeavor, and the mechanism responsible for reflux in singers is similar to that associated with reflux following other athletic activities, lifting, and other conditions that alter abdominal pressures such as pregnancy (which is also influenced by hormonal factors).

Second, many singers do not eat before performing because a full stomach interferes with abdominal support and promotes reflux. Performances usually take place at night. Consequently, the singer returns home hungry and eats a large meal before going to bed.

Third, performance careers are particularly stressful, a factor that may be associated with increased production of gastric acid. Fourth, many singers pay little attention to good nutrition, frequently consuming caffeine, fatty foods (including fast foods), spicy foods, citrus products (especially lemons), and tomatoes (including pizza and spaghetti sauce). In addition, because of the great demands singers place on their voices, even slight alterations caused by peptic mucositis of the larynx produce symptoms that may impair performance. Thus, singers are certainly more likely to seek care because of reflux symptoms than are individuals with fewer vocal demands. However, careful inquiry and physical examination reveal similar problems among all patients. Most of the voice problems associated with reflux laryngitis appear to be due to direct mucosal damage from proximal reflux. The effects of distal reflux alone on laryngeal function have not been studied.

Voice abnormalities and vocal fold pathology due to reflux of gastric juice onto the vocal folds may occur. Severe coughing may cause vocal fold hemorrhage or mucosal tears, sometimes leading to permanent dysphonia by causing scarring that obliterates the layers of the lamina propria and fixes the epithelium to deeper layers. Aspiration, caused by reflux, also makes reactive airway disease difficult to control. Even mild pulmonary obstruction impairs voice support. Consequently, afflicted patients subconsciously strain to compensate with muscles in the neck and throat, which are designed for delicate control, not for power source functions.[5,27] This behavior is typically responsible for vocal nodules and other lesions related to voice abuse. It also appears likely that some extra-esophageal symptoms of reflux are due to stimulation of the vagus nerve rather than (or in addition to) topical irritation. The role of vagal reflexes in reflux laryngitis remains to be clarified.

Posterior Laryngitis and Related Conditions

In addition to erythema and edema, more serious vocal fold pathology may be caused by reflux laryngitis. In 1968, Cherry and Margulies[28] recognized that reflux laryngitis might be a causative factor in contact ulcers and granulomas of the posterior portion of the vocal folds, conditions that we discuss in detail below. They also observed that treatment of peptic esophagitis resulted in resolution of vocal process granulomas. Delahunty and Cherry[29] followed up on this observation by applying gastric juice to the vocal processes of 2 dogs and applying saliva to the vocal processes of a third dog who was used as a control. The control dog's vocal folds remained normal; the other dogs developed granulomas at the sites of repeated acid application. The experiment by Delahunty and Cherry is particularly interesting. The posterior portion of the left vocal fold of 2 dogs was exposed to gastric acid for a total of only 20 minutes per day, 5 days out of every 7, for a total of 29 days of exposure in a 39-day period. A total of 20 minutes out of 24 hours may not seem like an extensive exposure period; however, erythema and edema were apparent in both dogs by the fourth day of the first week. At the beginning of the second week, the larynges appeared normal after the 2-day rest period. However, visible reaction was provoked within 2 days after application was resumed, and the vocal folds never regained normal appearance. Marked inflammation, thickening, and irregularities were apparent in both dogs by the fourth week, and epithelial slough at the site of acid contact occurred on day 29 in 1 dog and day 32 in the other. Granulation tissue appeared shortly thereafter. A similar procedure on a control animal was performed applying saliva to the vocal fold instead of gastric juice, and the vocal fold remained normal. This research suggests that even relatively short periods of acid exposure may cause substantial abnormalities in laryngeal mucosa. Since then, numerous authors have recognized the importance of reflux laryngitis as a causative factor in laryngeal ulcers and granulomas, including intubation granuloma.[1,2,27,28,30–36] In addition to its etiological involvement in intubation granuloma, reflux laryngitis has long been recognized as a contributing factor to posterior glottic stenosis, especially following intubation.[37] Olson has suggested that it may also be a causative factor in cricoarytenoid joint arthritis through chronic inflammation and ulceration, beginning on the mucosa and involving the synovial cricoarytenoid joint.[34] In addition to posterior glottic and supraglottic stenosis, subglottic stenosis has also been reported as a complication of reflux.[3,38]

Laryngeal Granulomas

Laryngeal granulomas are a particularly vexing problem for patients and their physicians. Granulomas, like contact ulcers of the larynx, usually occur on the posterior aspect of the vocal folds, often on or above the cartilaginous portion. They may be unilateral, although it is also common to see a sizeable granuloma on one side and a contact ulcer on the other. Patients with ulcers or granulomas may complain of pain (laryngeal or referred otalgia), a globus sensation, hoarseness, painful phonation, and occasionally hemoptysis. Surprisingly, even large granulomas are often asymptomatic. These benign lesions usually contain fibroblasts, collagenous fibers, proliferated capillaries, leukocysts, and sometimes ulceration. Although the term "granuloma" is universally accepted, these laryngeal lesions are actually not granulomas histopathologically, but rather chronic inflammatory lesions. However, granulomas and ulcers may mimick more serious lesions such as carcinoma, tuberculosis, and granular cell tumor. Consequently, the clinical diagnosis of laryngeal granuloma must always be made with caution and must be considered tentative until the patient has been followed over time and a good response to treatment has been observed.

Understanding the etiology of laryngeal ulcers and granulomas is essential to clinical evaluation and treatment. Traditionally, ulcers and granulomas in the region of the vocal processes have been associated with trauma, especially intubation injury. However, they are also seen in young, apparently healthy professional voice users with no history of intubation or obvious laryngeal injury. In fact, the vast majority of granulomas and ulcerations (probably even those from intubation) are caused or aggravated by laryngopharyngeal reflux disease. In some patients, muscular tension dysphonia producing forceful vocal process contact may be contributory or causal.

Evaluation of patients with laryngeal ulcers or granulomas begins with a comprehensive history and physical examination. In addition to elucidating specific voice complaints and their importance to the individual patient's life and profession, the history is designed to reveal otolaryngologic and systemic abnormalities that may have caused dysphonia. Special attention is paid to symptoms of voice abuse and of laryngopharyngeal reflux, as listed above. It must be remembered that reflux laryngitis is commonly *not* accompanied by pyrosis or dyspepsia. The history also specifically seeks symptoms consistent with asthma, including voice fatigue following extensive use. Exercise-induced asthma can be provoked by the exercise of voice use, and even mild reactive airway disease undermines the power source of the voice and may lead to compensatory muscular tension dysphonia and consequent laryngeal granuloma or ulcer. Inquiry also systematically investigates all body systems for evidence of other diseases that present with a laryngeal mass. It is important to include a psychological assessment. Excessive stress may lead to increased acid production and symptomatic reflux and to muscular tension dysphonia. In such cases, it is important to identify and treat the underlying stressor, as well as the symptomatic expressions of the stress.

Mirror examination usually reveals the presence of a granuloma or ulcer, but more sophisticated evaluation is invaluable. In the presence of suspected laryngeal granuloma or ulcer, the author (RTS) routinely performs strobovideolaryngoscopy using both flexible and rigid endoscopes. Flexible examination reveals patterns of phonation and is extremely helpful in identifying muscular tension dysphonia and determining phonatory behaviors associated with forceful adduction. Recent observations (Steven Zeitels, MD, personal communication, 1997) suggest that some granuloma patients have a vocal fold closure pattern with initial forceful vocal process contact. This implies an adduction strategy with lateral cricoarytenoid dominance, and this observation is important in the treatment of granulomas that are refractory to therapy or recur. Rigid laryngeal telescopic examination provides magnified, detailed information of the lesions under slow-motion light, allowing analysis of their composition (solid granulomas versus fluid-filled cysts) and their effects on phonation. This examination also permits assessment of other areas of the vocal folds to rule out separate lesions (eg, vocal fold scar) that may be the real cause of the patient's voice complaint.

Evaluation also includes at least formal assessment by a speech-language pathologist (SLP) skilled in voice evaluation and care. In the author's (RTS) center, objective voice analysis and a vocal stress assessment with a singing voice specialist (even with nonsingers) are also included. In addition to a laryngologist, SLP, and singing voice specialist, other members of the voice team are often used, depending on the patient's problems. Additional team members include an acting voice specialist, psychologist, otolaryngologic nurse clinician, and consulting pulmonologist, neurologist, gastroenterologist, and others. The information provided by these evaluations helps establish the degree to which voice abuse/misuse is present, and it guides the design of an individualized therapy plan.

Reflux must be suspected in virtually all cases of granuloma. It can be evaluated by 24-hour pH monitor, barium swallow with water siphonage (routine barium swallows are not satisfactory for diagnosing reflux, and the accuracy of barium swallow even with water siphonage is debatable), and/or a therapeutic trial of medical management. If there is historical evidence of prolonged reflux symptoms, formal gastroenterological evaluation to rule out Barrett's esophagus is often advisable. If a therapeutic trial of medications without confirmatory tests is elected, marked improvement in symptoms and signs should occur following daily use of a proton pump inhibitor (before breakfast and dinner) within 1 month.

Treatment for laryngopharyngeal reflux should be aggressive. The condition usually requires high doses of medication for prolonged periods (often a lifetime). We generally start with 20 mg of omeprazole twice daily, a liquid antacid or an H_2-blocker in addition to the proton pump inhibitor, sometimes a prokinetic agent, avoidance of eating for a few hours before going to sleep, elevation of the head of the bed, diet modification, and avoidance of caffeine or alcohol. A more individualized regimen can be designed following 24-hour pH monitor studies. For example, some singers reflux severely whenever they sing, but do not experience reflux at other times, even when they are supine. Consequently, lifestyle modifications may be individualized. The efficacy of oral steroids for treatment of laryngeal granulomas and ulcers has not been proven, but they are used commonly on the basis of anecdotal evidence, especially for granulomas and ulcers that appear acutely inflamed. For these conditions, low doses of steroids for longer periods are usually given, such as triamcinolone 4 mg twice a day for 3 weeks. Steroid inhalers are not recommended. They may lead to laryngitis, laryngeal *Candida* infections, and prolonged use may cause vocal fold atrophy.

At the end of 1 month of therapy including antireflux measures, voice therapy, and possibly steroids, substantial improvement in the appearance of the larynx should be seen. Ulcers should be healed, and granulomas should be substantially smaller. Repeated strobovideolaryngoscopy examinations allow comparison of lesion size over time. If such improvements are not noted, aggressive therapy and close follow-up can be continued until the mass lesion disappears or stabilizes.

If the mass does not disappear, or if response to the first month of aggressive therapy produces no substantial improvement, biopsy should be performed to rule out carcinoma and other possible causes. If the surgeon is reasonably certain that the lesion is a granuloma, injection of an aqueous steroid preparation into the base of the lesion at the time of surgery may be helpful. As long as a good specimen is obtained, the laser may be used for resection of suspected granulomas because the lesions are usually not on the vibratory margin, and they are often friable. However, the author usually uses traditional instruments, to avoid the third-degree burn caused by the laser (even with a microspot) in the treatment of this chronic, irritative condition.

It is essential that causative factors, especially reflux and voice abuse, be controlled strictly following laryngeal surgery. The patient is kept on optimal doses of a proton pump inhibitor prior to surgery and for at least 6 weeks following surgery. Surgeons should not hesitate to use omeprazole 20 mg as frequently as 4 times a day under these circumstances, if necessary. Following surgery, absolute voice rest (writing pad) is prescribed until the surgical area has remucosalized. This is usually approximately 1 week and virtually never longer than 10 to 14 days. There are no indications for prolonged absolute voice rest. Voice therapy is reinstituted on the day when phonation is resumed, and frequent short therapy sessions and close monitoring are maintained throughout the healing period.

As previously stated, granulomas recur in some patients. In all such cases, aggressive re-evaluation of reflux with 24-hour pH monitor studies is warranted. Often endoscopy and biopsy of esophageal and postcricoid mucosa is appropriate. Twenty-four hour pH monitor studies should be conducted not only off all medications, but also when the patient is taking a proton pump inhibitor or H_2-blocker. Some patients are resistant to omeprazole and will have normal acid secretions despite even 80 mg of omeprazole per day. In such patients, H_2-blockers may be preferable. When medical management is insufficient, laparoscopic fundoplication should be considered prior to repeated granuloma excisions. Voice use must also be optimized with the help of the speech-language pathologist and voice team, and the laryngologist must be sure that good vocal technique is carried over outside the medical office into the patient's daily life.

Occasionally patients may develop multiple recurrent granulomas even after excellent reflux control (including fundoplication), surgical removal including steroid injection into the base of the granulomas, and voice therapy. Medical causes other than reflux and muscular tension dysphonia must be ruled out, particularly granulomatous diseases including sarcoidosis and tuberculosis and neoplasm. Pathology slides from previous surgical procedures should be reviewed.

When it has been established that the recurrent lesions are typical granulomas occurring in the absence of laryngopharyngeal reflux, the cause is almost always phonatory trauma. When voice therapy has been insufficient to permit adequate healing, some of these uncommonly difficult patient problems can be solved by temporary paresis of selected vocal fold adductor muscles (particularly the lateral cricoarytenoid) using botulinum toxin injection. Although this treatment approach has been effective in a small number of cases, it is not recommended as initial therapy and is appropriate only for selected recalcitrant cases.

Carcinoma

It appears likely that acid reflux laryngitis may also be causally related to laryngeal carcinoma. The association of gastroesophageal reflux laryngitis disease with Barrett's esophagus and esophageal carcinoma has been well established. Delahunty biopsied the posterior laryngeal mucosa in a patient with reflux laryngitis and reported epithelial hyperplasia with parakeratosis and papillary down-growth.[4] Olson reported 5 patients (young, nonsmokers, nondrinkers) with posterior laryngeal carcinoma in whom he believed reflux to be a cofactor.[34] This issue was also addressed by Morrison.[39] Although the causal relationship between reflux and laryngeal cancer has not been established with absolute certainty, it appears probable.

Delayed Wound Healing

In addition to its possible carcinogenic potential, the chronic irritation of reflux laryngitis may be responsible for failure of wound healing. Reflux appears to delay the resolution not only of vocal process ulcers and granulomas, but also of healing following vocal fold surgery. For this reason, otolaryngologists are becoming increasingly aggressive about diagnosing and treating reflux before subjecting patients to vocal fold surgery, even for conditions unrelated to the reflux.

Sudden Infant Death Syndrome

Evidence suggests that sudden infant death syndrome (SIDS) may also be causally related to acid reflux into the larynx.[40] Hence, SIDS must join laryngeal and esophageal cancer at the top of the list of serious otolaryngologic consequences of reflux laryngitis. Wetmore investigated the effects of acid on the larynges of maturing rabbits by applying solutions of acid or saline at 15-day intervals up to 60 days of age.[40] Since the larynx is not only a site of resistance in the airway, but also contains the afferent limb for reflexes that regulate respiration, he discovered that acid exposure resulted in significant obstructive, central, and mixed apnea. Gasping respirations and frequent swallowing were observed as associated symptoms. Central apnea occurred in all age groups but had a peak incidence at 45 days. Acid-induced obstructive apnea in rabbits is similar to obstructive apnea previously recognized in human infants with gastroesophageal disease.[40,41] However, the demonstration of acid-induced central apnea produced by acid stimulation of the larynx is more ominous. Central apnea has been demonstrated in other animal models as a result of different forms of laryngeal stimulation. Central apnea resulting in fatal asphyxia has also been described in several animal models. Wetmore's study suggests that gastroesophageal reflux alone is capable of triggering fatal central apnea. This is particularly compelling when one recognizes that the peak incidence of central apnea occurring at 45 days in the rabbit corresponds well with the peak incidence of SIDS in humans, which occurs between 2 and 4 months of age.

CONCLUSION

Treatment considerations in reflux patients are discussed in greater detail in Chapters 7 and 8. However, it should be emphasized that patients with reflux laryngitis frequently require more intensive therapy with higher doses of H_2-blockers or earlier use of proton pump inhibitors than patients with dyspepsia in the absence of laryngeal symptoms and signs. In addition to monitoring symptoms and signs of reflux laryngitis, response to treatment is best judged by combined intra-esophageal and intragastric pH monitoring of patients while they are receiving treatment. Such studies are worthwhile even when patients are taking proton pump inhibitors, since some patients are omeprazole-resistent.[42,43] Our recent observations suggest that omeprazole resistance also can develop in patients who initially respond well to the medication. Moreover, it must be recognized that a normal pH 24-hour monitor study does not indicate the absence of reflux. Rather, it demonstrates the absence of *acid* reflux. Reflux of pH-neutral liquid may still be present and may produce symptoms, especially in singers and actors. Study of this phenomenon and its optimal management is badly needed. At the present time, it seems likely that we may conclude that surgical correction of reflux is appropriate in a higher percentage of patients, especially considering the efficacy and decreased morbidity associated with laparoscopic fundoplication and the potential costs and risks associated with the use of H_2-blockers or omeprazole for periods of many years. Research into appropriate treatment regimens is ongoing, and extensive additional investigation on the consequences of reflux on the larynx and on all of the other mucosal surfaces above the cricopharyngeus muscle is needed.

REFERENCES

1. Johnson LF. New concepts and methods in the study and treatment of gastroesophageal reflux disease. *Med Clin North Am.* 1981;65:1195–1222.
2. Ward PH, Zwitman D, Hanson D, et al. Contact ulcers and granulomas of the larynx: new insights into their etiology as a basis for more rational treatment. *Otolaryngol Head Neck Surg.* 1980;88:262–269.
3. Bain WM, Harrington JR, Thomas LE, et al. Head and neck manifestations of gastroesophageal reflux. *Laryngoscope.* 1983;93:175–179.
4. Delahunty JE. Acid laryngitis. *J Laryngol Otol.* 1972;86:335–342.
5. Sataloff RT. The human voice. *Sci Am.* 1993;267:108–115.
6. Sataloff RT. Professional singers: the science and art of clinical care. *Am J Otolaryngol.* 1981;8:251–266.
7. Sataloff RT. Reflux and other gastroenterologic conditions that may affect the voice. In: Sataloff RT, *Professional Voice: The Science and Art of Clinical Care.* 2nd ed. San Diego, Calif: Singular Publishing Group; 1997:3
8. Chodosh P. Gastro-esophago-pharyngeal reflux. *Laryngoscope.* 1977;87:1418–1427.
9. Hallewell JD, Cole TB. Isolated head and neck symptoms due to hiatus hernia. *Arch Otolaryngol.* 1970;92:499–501.
10. Ward PH, Berci G. Observations on the pathogenesis of chronic nonspecific pharyngitis and laryngitis. *Laryngoscope.* 1982;92:1377–1382.
11. Olson NR. The problem of gastroesophageal reflux. *Otolaryngol Clin North Am.* 1986;19:119–133.
12. Ossakow SJ, Elta G, Colturi T, Bogdassarian R, Nostrant TT. Esophageal reflux and dysmotility as the basis for persistent cervical symptoms. *Ann Otol Rhinol Laryngol.* 1987;96:387–392.
13. Kuriloff DB, Chodosh P, Goldfarb R, Ongseng F. Detection of gastroesophageal reflux in the head and neck: the role of scintigraphy. *Ann Otol Rhinol Laryngol.* 1989;98:74–80.
14. Lumpkin SMM, Bishop SG, Katz PO. Chronic dysphonia secondary to gastroesophageal reflux disease (GERD): diagnosis using simultaneous dual-probe prolonged pH monitoring. *J Voice.* 1989;3:351–355.
15. McNally PR, Maydonovitch CL, Prosek RA, Collette RP, Wong RKH. Evaluation of gastroesophageal reflux as a cause of idiopathic hoarseness. *Digest Dis Sci.* 1989;34:1900–1904.
16. Wiener GJ, Koufman JA, Wu WC, Cooper JB, Richter JE, Castell DO. Chronic hoarseness secondary to gastroesophageal reflux disease: documentation with 24-hr ambulatory pH monitoring. *Amer J Gastroenterol.* 1989;84:1503–1507.
17. Katz PO. Ambulatory esophageal and hypopharyngeal pH monitoring in patients with hoarseness. *Am J Gastroenterol.* 1990;85:38–40.

18. Freeland AP, Ardran GM, Emrys-Roberts E. Globus hystericus and reflux oesophagitis. *J Laryngol Otol.* 1974;88:1025–1031.
19. Koufman JA. Otolaryngologic manifestations of gastroesophageal reflux disease (GERD): a clinical investigation of 225 patients using ambulatory 24-hr pH monitoring and an experimental investigation of the role of acid and pepsin in the development of laryngeal injury. *Laryngoscope.* 1991;101(suppl 53, pt 2).
20. Pesce G, Caligaris F. Le laringiti posteriori nella pathologia dell'apparato digerente. *Arch Ital Laryngol.* 1966;74:77–92.
21. Vaughan CW, Strong MS. Medical management of organic laryngeal disorders. *Otolaryngol Clin North Am.* 1984;17:705–712.
22. Barkin RL, Stein ZL. GE reflux and vocal pitch. *Hosp Pract.* 1989;24:20.
23. Kambic V, Radsel Z. Acid posterior laryngitis: aetiology, histology, diagnosis and treatment. *J Laryngol Otol.* 1984;98:1237–1240.
24. Jacob P, Kahrilas PJ, Herzon G. Proximal esophageal pH-metry in patients with reflux laryngitis. *Gastroenterology.* 1991;100:305–310.
25. Wilson JA, White A, von Haacke NP, Maran AG, Heading RC, Pryde A, Piris J. Gastroesophageal reflux and posterior laryngitis. *Ann Otol Rhinol Laryngol.* 1989;98:405–410.
26. Sataloff RT. *Professional Voice: The Science and Art of Clinical Care.* 2nd ed. San Diego, Calif: Singular Publishing Group, Inc; 1997:735–753, 765–774.
27. Sataloff RT. *Professional Voice: The Science and Art of Clinical Care,* 2nd ed. San Diego, CA: Singular Publishing Group, Inc. 1997.
28. Cherry J, Margulies S. Contact Ulcer of the Larynx. *Laryngoscope.* 1968;78:1937–1940.
29. Delahunty JE, Cherry J. Experimentally produced vocal cord granulomas. *Laryngoscope.* 1968;78:1941–1947.
30. Gould WJ, Sataloff RT, Spiegel JR. *Voice Surgery.* St. Louis, Mo: CV Mosby Co; 1993.
31. Cherry J, Siegal C, Margulies S, et al. Pharyngeal localization of symptoms of gastroesophageal reflux. *Ann Otol Rhinol Laryngol.* 1970;79:912–915.
32. Goldberg M, Noyek A, Pritzker KPH. Laryngeal granuloma secondary to gastroesophageal reflux. *J Otolaryngol.* 1978;7:196–202.
33. Ohman L, Tibbling L, Olafsson J, et al. Esophageal dysfunction in patients with contact ulcer of the larynx. *Ann Otol Rhinol Laryngol.* 1983;92:228–230.
34. Olson NR. Effects of stomach acid on the larynx. *Proc Am Laryngol Assoc.* 1983;104:108–112.
35. Teisanu E, Hecioia D, Dimitriu T, Calarasu R, Marinescu A. Tulburari Faringolaringiene la Bolnavii cu reflux gastroesofagian. *Otorinolaringologia.* 1978;23:279–286.
36. Miko TL. Peptic (contact ulcer) granuloma of the larynx. *J Clin Pathol.* 1989;42:800–804.
37. Bogdassarian RS, Olson NR. Posterior glottic laryngeal stenosis. *Otolaryngol Head Neck Surg.* 1980;88:765–772.
38. Fligny I, Francois M, Algrain Y, Polonovski JM, Contencin P, Narcy P. Subglottic stenosis and gastroesophageal reflux [Stenoses sous-glottiquee et refluxgastro-oesophagien]. *Ann Otolaryngol Chir Cervicofac.* 1989;106:193–196.

39. Morrison M. Is chronic gastroesophageal reflux a causative factor in glottic carcinoma? *Otolaryngol Head Neck Surg.* 1988;99:370–373.
40. Wetmore RP. The effects of acid upon the larynx of the maturing rabbit and their possible significance to sudden infant death syndrome. *Laryngoscope.* 1993;103:1242–1254.
41. Spitzer GR, Boyle JT, Tuchman DN, et al. Awake apnea associated with gastroesophageal reflux: a specific clinical syndrome. *J Pediatr.* 1984;104: 200–205.
42. Bough ID, Castell DO, Sataloff RT, Hills JR. Gastroesophageal reflux disease resistant to omeprazole therapy. *J Voice.* 1995;9:205–211.
43. Klinkenberg-Knol EC, Meuwissen GSM. Combined gastric and oesophageal 24-hour pH monitoring and oesophageal manometry in patients with reflux disease, resistent to treatment with omeprazole. *Aliment Pharmacol Ther.* 1990;4:485–495.

CHAPTER

Diagnostic Tests for Gastroesophageal Reflux

The diagnosis of gastroesophageal reflux (GERD) is normally based on a combination of the history, appropriate diagnostic tests, and relief of symptoms with carefully selected antireflux therapy. The patient presenting to the otolaryngologist poses special problems because the typical symptoms of reflux, heartburn, and regurgitation are often absent, When used appropriately, diagnostic testing with barium radiographs, esophagoscopy, laryngoscopy, esophageal motility testing, and/or ambulatory pH monitoring allows the clinician to demonstrate that reflux occurs, identify the end-organ effects of reflux including esophagitis or laryngitis, confirm that symptoms are due to reflux, and evaluate the effects of reflux on LES pressure and esophageal clearance. The approach to diagnosis of laryngopharyngeal reflux in a general or otolaryngologic practice includes careful physical examination, judicious use of a therapeutic trial of antireflux therapy, and diagnostic testing. This chapter discusses the use of each of these modalities in GERD in general, with specific reference to the otolaryngologic patient (Table 6-1).

THERAPEUTIC TRIAL

When a patient presents with typical heartburn and regurgitation, diagnostic studies are usually not needed. Relief of symptoms after a

TABLE 6-1. *Diagnostic Tests for Gastroesphageal Reflux*

Is reflux present?
Barium swallow
pH monitoring

Is there mucosal injury?
Barium swallow (air contrast) study
Endoscopy
Mucosal biopsy

Are symptoms due to reflux?
Therapeutic trial
pH monitoring (with symptom index)

Can prognostic or preoperative information be obtained?
Esophageal manometry
pH monitoring

therapeutic trial with H_2-antagonists, prokinetic agents, or proton pump inhibitors for 8 weeks can confirm that the symptoms are secondary to GERD. Since heartburn is often absent in the otolaryngologic patient, the end-point of the therapeutic trial is dependent on other presenting symptoms; and diagnostic tests are more often necessary to confirm the diagnosis. Historical clues that otolaryngologic symptoms may be due to GERD such as morning hoarseness, halitosis, excess phlegm, dry mouth, throat clearing, and others have been discussed in previous chapters.

If a therapeutic trial is used in the patient with suspected GERD and otolaryngologic symptoms, higher doses of antireflux therapy, usually with a proton pump inhibitor, for longer periods of time are needed. However, neither cost effectiveness nor clinical efficacy of any medical regimen has been tested. We currently use a proton pump inhibitor (omeprazole or lansoprazole) twice a day for a minimum of 8 to 12 weeks as a therapeutic trial for laryngeal symptoms suspected due to GERD. (see Approach to the Patient, below)

BARIUM RADIOGRAPHS

Barium studies are relatively inexpensive and widely available for use in diagnosis of esophageal disease. When evaluating the esophagus a double contrast barium swallow is needed for optimal evaluation. An upper GI series usually results in insufficient evaluation of esophageal function, concentrates excessively on the stomach and duodenum, and does not give enough attention to potential mucosal or motility abnormalities in the esophagus. A hiatal hernia is the most common abnormality seen on barium swallow. However, up to 60% of the adult population will have a hernia,[1] making this a nonspecific finding and not diagnostic of GERD. Free reflux is seen in up to 30% of normal patients and may be absent in up to 60% of patients with GERD established by pH monitoring,[2] making the barium study an insensitive and nonspecific study for GERD. It has been suggested that reflux of barium to or above the carina or to the thoracic inlet is indicative of the potential for aspiration and is useful as an aid in the diagnosis of GERD associated laryngitis. There are no prospective or controlled studies to substantiate this clinical impression. This finding is usually reported with the patient in the supine position, making this observation of little use. This so-called "high" reflux on a barium study has not been well correlated with proximal acid exposure on ambulatory pH monitoring. The use of barium swallow with water siphonage has been used to aid in diagnosis of reflux in the otolaryngology patient. Occasionally patients will show abnormalities on barium swallow with water siphonage, which are interpreted as confirming a diagnosis of pathologic reflux. This should be done with caution as the true positive predictive value has not been studied. In professional singers and actors, especially, barium swallow with water siphonage does, however, provide a good clinical approximation of daily activities. To optimize mucosal function, it is essential for singers and actors to remain well hydrated. Consequently they drink large amounts of water, routinely carry water bottles with them, and drink substantial quantities shortly before they sing. This routine behavior is similar to the water siphon portion of the barium swallow, which raises the question of whether positive water siphonage tests may provide useful information, at least in professional voice users, even when a 24-hour pH monitor study is normal. It is important that this test be performed with the patient in the upright position. Specific mucosal abnormalities on double contrast barium studies, such as thickening of esophageal mucosal folds, erosions, or esophageal ulcers, are seen in a minority of patients with GERD, making this study relatively insensitive for this diagnosis. The diagnosis of Barrett's esophagus is rarely made conclusively by a barium swallow.

    The optimal use of the barium study is to evaluate patients with suspected complications of GERD such as motility abnormalities or peptic stricture, abnormalities seen in patients with accompanying solid and/or liquid dysphagia. A barium swallow can identify rings, webs, or other obstructive lesions including carcinoma that are seen in patients with dysphagia, but these are unusual complications of GERD. A solid bolus such as a marshmallow or a barium cookie can be given to help localize the site of obstruction in a patient with solid dysphagia.

Although the barium swallow allows demonstration that reflux is occurring and can demonstrate mucosal injury, it is rarely of value in establishing a diagnosis of GERD. Its best use is in evaluation of the patient with dysphagia and it should be performed in conjunction with endoscopy in these patients. Additionally, no prospective studies have been done with barium swallow in patients with GERD and laryngitis.

RADIONUCLEOTIDE STUDIES

Scintigraphic studies have been suggested by a few investigations to be valuable in diagnosis of GERD. A radioisotope (Technetium 99 m-sulfur colloid) marker is mixed with a measured quantity of liquid (usually H_2O) and graded abdominal compression is used to unmask reflux. Originally proposed as a sensitive test its reliability has been questioned and is no longer considered a useful investigation.[3]

ENDOSCOPY

Endoscopy is used to document mucosal disease and establish a diagnosis of erosive esophagitis or Barrett's metaplasia. When patients with frequent heartburn and regurgitation are studied prospectively, erosive esophagitis is seen in 45% to 60% of patients.[4] The others will have nonerosive disease (mucosal edema, hyperemia, or a normal-appearing esophagus). Erosive esophagitis suggests a serious form of GERD in which patients require continuous medical therapy with a proton pump inhibitor or antireflux surgery for effective symptom relief and healing. Barrett's esophagus is seen in 10% to 15% of reflux patients undergoing endoscopy.[5] Unfortunately, there is no classic presentation of Barrett's esophagus. However, it is most common in white males over 50 years of age.

Erosive esophagitis is extremely rare in patients with extraesophageal symptoms. Although 50% of patients with unexplained chest pain and normal coronary arteries have GERD, the prevalence of erosive esophagitis is 10% or less.[6] In GERD associated asthma, endoscopic esophagitis has been reported in 30% to 40% of adult patients.[7,8] In patients with laryngitis, erosive esophagitis is seen in only 20% to 30%, making this study rarely diagnostic of GERD.[9,10]

There are no absolute indications for endoscopy in the patient with suspected GERD. In general, endoscopy is performed in patients who do not respond to a therapeutic trial of medical therapy, patients with symptoms for greater than 5 years to rule out Barrett's metaplasia, and patients with the "alarm" symptoms of dysphagia, odynophagia, weight loss, anemia, or gastrointestinal bleeding.[11]

Endoscopic findings may help predict the prognosis and outcome of medical therapy. Patients with erosive esophagitis will almost always require long-term proton pump inhibitor therapy for healing and symptom relief. Recurrence of erosive esophagitis is seen in up to 80% of patients within 3 to 6 months following discontinuation of medications[12]; these patients usually require continuous pharmacologic therapy for effective long-term control. Because patients with nonerosive esophagitis seldom progress to more severe forms of esophagitis, they can be managed with a range of pharmacologic treatments. Endoscopy is useful for long-term treatment planning in difficult-to-manage cases.

Given the rarity of erosive esophagitis, we do not routinely use endoscopy as the initial study in patients with suspected GERD-related otolaryngologic disease, chest pain, asthma, or cough, preferring ambulatory pH monitoring or a therapeutic trial as the initial diagnostic test (see below). If GERD is confirmed and long-term medical therapy (or antireflux surgery) is needed, we consider endoscopy to rule out Barrett's esophagus.

ESOPHAGEAL BIOPSY

Biopsy and cytology are of limited value in evaluation of the patient with GERD unless Barrett's esophagus or malignancy is suspected. The light microscopic signs of GERD—elongation of rete pegs and hyperplasia of the basal cell layer[13]—do not distinguish between acute and chronic disease and do not help predict response to therapy. The microscopic signs of active esophagitis, polymorphonuclear leukocytes and eosinophils, are seen in a minority of adult patients,[13] so they are insensitive diagnostic findings. Biopsy may be more useful in the pediatric population where a higher frequency of these findings has been reported.[14] The author only biopsies the esophagus in patients with GERD in whom Barrett's metaplasia or malignancy is suspected. Mucosa that appears normal endoscopically is not biopsied.

If Barrett's metaplasia is suspected, a systematic biopsy protocol should be followed to confirm the diagnosis and rule out dyplasia or carcinoma.[15] Endoscopic surveillance with biopsies to rule out dysplasia every 1 to 2 years is the current standard of practice for management of patients with Barrett's.[15]

PROLONGED AMBULATORY pH MONITORING

Prolonged pH monitoring is the most important study to quantify esophageal reflux and determine whether symptoms are related to GERD. The study is performed by placing a 2-mm diameter antimony catheter transnasally into the distal esophagus with an electrode placed 5 cm above the lower esophageal sphincter, which is identified by esophageal manometry (Fig 6-1). The probe is connected to a small microcomputer that is worn on a belt or clipped to the waist so that the patient can be monitored in an ambulatory setting. Activity can be tailored to provoke reflux in the setting in which symptoms are normally produced. For example, a patient with chronic hoarseness who sings professionally will be reminded to sing during the study.

Multiple electrodes can be placed on a single catheter to monitor intragastric and intraesophageal pH, distal esophageal and proximal esophageal acid exposure, or all three simultaneously. Abnormal acid exposure in the proximal esophagus, just below the upper esophageal sphincter, predicts the potential for aspiration in patients with otolaryngologic symptoms. An intragastric electrode allows monitoring of the gastric acid response to antireflux therapy. Several investigators

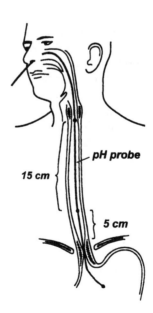

FIG 6-1. Illustrates dual channel antimony pH probe with electrodes 15 cm apart. Distal electrode is placed 5 cm above the lower esophageal sphincter. Proximal electrode is 20 cm above the lower sphincter just below the upper esophageal sphincter.

have placed probes above the upper esophageal sphincter in the hypopharynx[10,16] to document reflux above the UES, thus being more certain of aspiration as the cause of symptoms. Unfortunately, this placement creates difficulty in standardizing the distance between the proximal and distal probes and causes difficulty in placement of the distal esophageal probe 5 cm above the LES, the standard for developing normal values. Probes in the hypopharynx can be uncomfortable, normal values are not available, and are occasionally subject to interpretation error, including incorrect diagnosis of reflux due to probe drying, food or liquid ingestion, or other artifact resulting in a drop of pH <4 that is not a true reflux episode. If these technical problems can be resolved, placement above the UES would be ideal. At present normal values for distal reflux at 5 cm above the lower esophageal sphincter and for proximal reflux 20 cm above the sphincter are available, making this a more useful standard.[17,18] Normal values vary slightly between laboratories and should be included with reports from the laboratory performing the procedure. The microcomputer (data logger) has a symptom button that allows recording of up to 6 symptoms during a single study. The patient is asked to push the appropriate symptom button as well as to record symptoms on a diary card. This allows correlation of reflux events with symptoms, which is especially valuable in patients with asthma, cough, and chest pain and allows correlation between heartburn and reflux in patients who have continued symptoms on medical therapy. Symptom correlation in the otolaryngologic patient may be more difficult on a single study, particularly when symptoms are continuous and not produced by a single reflux episode. This is more likely in patients with laryngitis or chronic sore throat. Other symptoms such as throat clearing, cough, or symptoms provoked by singing may be correlated with single reflux episodes.

Prolonged pH monitoring is used in patients with heartburn to establish a diagnosis when symptoms have not responded to a trial of antireflux therapy and endoscopy is negative. In this case, a single channel pH probe can be placed with the distal probe 5 cm above the lower esophageal sphincter. Symptoms are correlated with reflux and reflux frequency is assessed. Patients with known GERD who have heartburn and regurgitation not responding to medical therapy can be monitored while still on therapy with a dual channel intragastric and distal esophageal probe to assess the adequacy of gastric acid suppression, esophageal reflux frequency, and to correlate symptoms with reflux events. Patients with continued esophageal acid exposure and/or symptoms may require additional therapy.

Patients with otolaryngologic symptoms, or other upper airway symptoms suggestive of GERD, are ideal candidates for prolonged ambulatory pH monitoring. We prefer performing monitoring early in the clinical course to establish a diagnosis and symptom correlation when possible. Dual channel pH monitoring with one electrode 5 cm above the LES and a second probe 20 cm above in the proximal esophagus just below the UES (Fig 6-1) is the procedure of choice. Abnormal distal esophageal acid exposure can be documented, establishing a diagnosis of GERD. Abnormal proximal reflux can be demonstrated, suggesting the potential for aspiration and lending stronger probability that the otolaryngologic symptom is due to GERD. If symptom correlation can be demonstrated, this will establish the diagnosis. The presence of proximal reflux appears to predict the response to medical therapy in patients with pulmonary disease.[19,20] This is less clear in the otolaryngologic patient. A small percentage of patients will have normal percent time of distal esophageal acid exposure, but demonstrable increased frequency of proximal reflux or reflux into the hypopharynx. This is seen in up to 30% of patients with otolaryngologic symptoms. In one study of 10 patients with reflux laryngitis, 3 of 10 (30%) demonstrated hypopharyngeal reflux with normal distal acid exposure.[16] In a larger, retrospective series of patients with pulmonary disease, 12% of patients reviewed had only abnormal proximal reflux[19]—a group that would have been diagnosed incorrectly as normal had only a single channel study been performed. These patients should be considered abnormal and treated aggressively.

Studies in adults with a variety of otolaryngologic symptoms demonstrate abnormal amounts of acid reflux in up to 75% of patients.[10] Abnormal acid exposure has been documented in upright and supine positions, although upright reflux seems more common. Ambulatory pH monitoring is most useful in assessing response to antireflux therapy, particularly in the patient who has failed to respond to a therapeutic trial of a proton pump inhibitor twice daily for 8 to 12 weeks. Intragastric, distal esophageal, and proximal esophageal pH can be monitored while therapy is continued. Adequacy of intragastric acid suppression can be assessed, as can the presence of esophageal acid exposure and correlation between reflux events and symptoms. This study is particularly valuable in patients who do not respond (or are resistant) to proton pump inhibitors. If acid reflux is still present, treatment can be increased or modified. If adequate acid suppression is achieved and symptoms persist, alternative diagnosis can be sought.

An area of some controversy is the evaluation of the patient with continued symptoms but no esophageal acid exposure on 24-hour pH monitoring. This is when a question of alkaline or pH neutral reflux may be raised. Current pH monitoring technology makes it possible to detect bilirubin pigment (bile) by use of a bilitec probe in addition to standard 24-hour pH monitoring. However, current data using this technique suggest that esophageal bile reflux rarely, if ever, occurs in the absence of acid reflux, making the bilitec probe useful only in select patients (see approach, below). The diagnosis of alkaline reflux should not be made based solely on the rise in pH above 7; careful analysis of pH rises above 7 coupled with symptom correlation may suggest alkaline reflux but are rarely if ever conclusively made with pH testing. The decision to proceed with surgical management for the suspicion of alkaline or pH neutral reflux is a clinical one and must be made after careful consultation. Current pH technology cannot make this diagnosis.

ESOPHAGEAL MANOMETRY

Manometry will establish abnormal LES pressure or esophageal motility and is necessary preoperatively to evaluate contraction amplitude in the esophageal body. A single measurement of LES pressure is rarely low in patients with GERD. In the author's experience, only 4% of patients with gastroesophageal reflux disease have a low LES pressure.[21] Esophageal motility abnormalities are found more frequently. The most common finding appears to be ineffective esophageal motility (IEM) (amplitude of contraction in the distal esophagus less than 30 mm Hg occurring with 30% or more of water swallows). In the author's experience, this is the most common abnormality in patients with GERD, seen in approximately 35% of patients with esophagitis.[21] IEM appears more common in GERD-related laryngitis, asthma, and cough.[22] Esophageal manometry is performed prior to antireflux surgery to establish the presence or absence of ineffective esophageal motility. The surgeon will usually perform a Nissen fundoplication (360° wrap) in patients with normal peristalsis and a Toupet procedure (240° wrap) in patients with IEM. Patients with IEM and respiratory symptoms do not appear to respond as well to antireflux surgery if respiratory complaints are the presenting symptom.

HIATAL HERNIA

A hiatal hernia is not predictive of reflux as a cause of the patients' symptoms. Up to 60% of patients over the age of 60 will demonstrate a hiatal hernia identified on barium swallow examination. One study suggested that only 9% of patients with a radiographically demonstrated hernia will actually have typical reflux symptoms.[23]

Hernias do change the relationship of the LES and crural diaphragm. The LES is displaced above the diaphragm. The low pressure in the hernia can act as a reservoir for acid, allowing earlier reflux during LES relaxations and may delay esophageal clearance.[24] Patients with large hernias who also have low LES pressure may be more prone to reflux[25] if changes occur in intra-abdominal pressure.

APPROACH TO THE PATIENT WITH GERD-RELATED OTOLARYNGOLOGIC ABNORMALITIES

In patients with GERD-related complaints, a thorough history, physical examination, and laryngoscopy should be performed (Fig 6-2). If dysphagia is present, a videoendoscopic swallowing evaluation should be considered and a barium swallow should be ordered to rule out stricture disease or motility abnormalities. The clinician's dilemma revolves around the choice of early diagnostic testing with prolonged pH monitoring or institution of a therapeutic trial. The "best" approach is not clear. Although diagnostic testing with ambulatory pH monitoring would be ideal, there are several limitations: (1) pH monitoring is

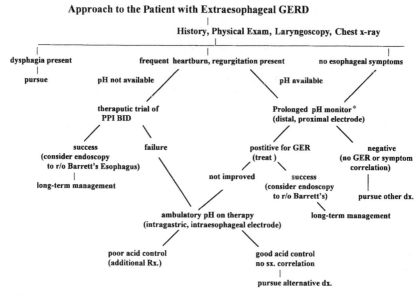

*If pH monitor is not available or clinical suspicion is high despite no esophageal symptoms, a therapeutic trial is a reasonable first intervention.

FIG 6-2. Outline of approach to the patient with gastroesophageal reflux disease and otolaryngologic disease. (PPI = proton pump inhibitor; GER = gastroesophageal reflux; BID = twice daily)

not always available. (2) The sensitivity and specificity are clearly not 100%. (3) Patients do not reflux with the same frequency every day. (4) Variability in both distal and proximal esophageal acid exposure time in patients with extraesophageal GERD is common, increasing the possibility of a false negative pH study if physiologic acid exposure is seen on a single study.

If the history and laryngoscopic examination raise high clinical suspicion of GERD, if prolonged monitoring is not available, if frequent heartburn and regurgitation are present, or if there is endoscopic documentation of GERD, a therapeutic trial of antireflux therapy is a reasonable initial choice. A recent study with empiric Omeprazole 40 mg at bedtime in patients with suspected reflux laryngitis found a 67% response in patients with laryngeal symptoms suggestive of GERD.[27] Another study found 70% success with empiric Omeprazole 20 mg BID for a similar time period.[28] We use a trial of proton pump inhibitor twice daily in combination with dietary and behavior modification (omeprazole 20 mg or lansoprazole 30 mg BID) for 8 to 12 weeks. If the patient does not respond, pH monitoring should be performed while proton pump inhibitor therapy is continued.[30] A dual channel probe with intragastric and distal esophageal electrodes should be placed to ascertain adequate gastric acid suppression and to assess the presence of esophageal acid exposure. If distal esophageal acid exposure is seen more than 1.2% of the time, this is definitely abnormal and additional medical therapy is indicated.[29] "Normal" esophageal acid exposure, particularly when any proximal esophageal acid exposure is documented, may not always be a negative study. A positive symptom index may be seen occasionally even in patients with "normal" distal acid exposure; and this, too, is abnormal and warrants additional therapy. The *absence* of any esophageal acid exposure and adequate gastric acid suppression (pH >4, 50% of total time) suggests adequate medical therapy and an alternative diagnosis should be pursued. If GERD-associated otolaryngologic disease is documented, endoscopy is indicated in many cases to rule out Barrett's esophagus prior to long-term medical therapy or surgery.

REFERENCES

1. Ott DJ, Wu WC, Gelfand DW. Reflux esophagitis revisited: prospective analysis of radiologic accuracy. *Gastrointest Radiol.* 1981;6:1–7.
2. Richter JE, Castell DO. Gastroesophageal reflux: pathogenesis, diagnosis, and therapy. *Ann Intern Med.* 1982;97:93–103.
3. Bough D, Sataloff RT, Castell DO, Hills JR, Gideon RM, Spiegel JR. Gastroesophageal reflux resistant to omeprazole therapy. *J Voice.* 1995;9:205–211.

4. Jenkins AF, Cowan RJ, Richter JE. Gastroesophageal scintigraphy: is it a sensitive test for gastroesophageal reflux disease? *J Clin Gastroenterol.* 1985;7:127.
5. Winters C, Spurling TJ, Chobanian SJ, et al. Barrett's esophagus: a prevalent, occult complication of gastroesophageal reflux disease. *Gastroenterology.* 1987; 92:118–123.
6. Lieberman DA, Oehlke M, Helfand M, et al. Risk factors for Barrett's esophagus in community based practice. *Am J Gastroenterol.* 1997;92: 1293–1297.
7. Cherian P, Smith LF, Bardham KD, Thorpe J, Oakley GD, Dawson D. Esophageal tests in the evaluation of non-cardiac chest pain. *Dis Esophagus.* 1995;8:129–133.
8. Harding SM, Guzzo MR, Richter JE. Prevalence of GERD in asthmatics without reflux symptoms. *Gastroenterology.* 1997;4:A141.
9. Sontag SJ, O'Connell S, Khandelwal S, et al. Most asthmatics have gastroesophageal reflux with or without bronchodilator therapy. *Gastroenterology.* 1990;99:613–618.
10. Weiner GJ, Kaufman JA, Wu WC, et al. Chronic hoarseness secondary to gastroesophageal reflux disease. *Am J Gastroenterol.* 1989;84:503–508.
11. Koufman JA. The otolaryngologic manifestations of gastroesophageal reflux disease: a clinical investigation of 225 patients using ambulatory 24-hour pH monitoring and an experimental investigation of the role of acid and pepsin in the development of laryngeal injury. *Laryngoscope.* 1991:101:1.
12. DeVault KR, Castell DO. Guidelines for the diagnosis and treatment of gastroesophageal reflux disease. *Arch Intern Med.* 1995;155:2165–2173.
13. Hetzel D, Dent J, Reed W, et al. Healing and relapse of severe peptic esophagitis after treatment with Omeprazole. *Gastroenterology.* 1988;95: 903–912.
14. Imail-Beigi F, Horton PF, Pope CE. Histological consequences of gastroesophageal reflux in man. *Gastroenterology.* 1970;58:163–174.
15. Winter CS, et al. Intraepithelial eosinophils: a new diagnostic criterion for reflux esophagitis. *Gastroenterology.* 1982;83:818.
16. Spechler SJ. Complications of gastroesophageal reflux disease. In: Castell DO, ed. *The esophagus.* Boston, Mass: Little Brown & Co; 1995:533-546.
17. Katz PO. Ambulatory esophageal and hypopharyngeal pH monitoring in patients with hoarseness. *Am J Gastroenterol.* 1990;85:38.
18. Johnson LF, DeMeester T. Twenty-four hour pH monitoring of the distal esophagus. *Am J Gastroenterol.* 1974;62:325–333.
19. Dobhan R, Castell DO. Normal and abnormal proximal esophageal acid exposure: results of ambulatory dual probe pH monitoring. *Am J Gastroenterol.* 1993;88:25–29.
20. Schnatz PF, Castell JA, Castell DO. Pulmonary symptoms associated with gastroesophageal reflux: use of ambulatory pH monitoring to diagnose and to direct therapy. *Am J Gastroenterol.* 1996;91:1715–1718.
21. Harding SM, Richter JE, Guzzo MR, et al. Asthma and gastroesophageal reflux: acid suppressive therapy improves asthma outcome. *Am J Med.* 1996;100:395–405.

22. Barrett J. Peghini P, Katz P, Castell J, Castell D. Ineffective esophageal motility (IEM): the most common manometric abnormality in GERD. *Gastroenterology*. 1997;112:Abstract 66.
23. Fouad YM, Koury R, Hatlebakk JG, Katz PO, Castell DO. Ineffective esophageal motility (IEM) is more prevalent in reflux patients with respiratory symptoms. *Gastroenterology*. 1998;114:Abstract 6506.
24. Palmer ED. The hiatus-esophagitis-esophageal stricture complex. Twenty year prospective study. *Am J Med*. 1968;44:566-572.
25. Sloan S, Kakrilas PJ. Impairment of esophageal emptying with hiatal hernia. *Gastroenterology*. 1991;100:596–605.
26. Sloan S, Rademaker AW, Kahrilas PJ. Determinants of gastroesophageal junction incompetence: hiatal hernia, lower esophageal sphincter, or both? *Ann Intern Med*. 1992;117:977–982.
27. Weiner GJ, Richter JE, Cooper JB, et al. The symptom index: a clinically important parameter of ambulatory 24-hour esophageal pH monitoring. *Am J Gastroenterol*. 1988;38:58–61.
28. Wo JM, Grist WJ, Gussack G, Delguardo JM, Waring JP. Empiric trial of high dose omeprazole in patients with posterior laryngitis: a prospective study. *Am J Gastroenterol*. 1997;92:2160–2165.
29. Metz DC, Childs ML, Ruiz C, Weinstein GS. Pilot study of the oral omeprazole test for reflux laryngitis. *Otolaryngol Head Neck Surg*. 1997;16:41–46.
30. Kuo B, Castell DO. Optimal dosing of omeprazole 40 mg daily: effects on gastric and esophageal pH and serum gastrin in healthy controls. *Am J Gastroenterol*. 1996;91:1532–1538.

CHAPTER

7

Behavioral and Medical Management of Gastroesophageal Reflux Disease

Gastroesophageal reflux disease (GERD) is a chronic relapsing condition with a variety of symptom presentations caused by the reflux of gastric contents—principally acid and pepsin—into the esophagus or beyond. Treatment of the patient with GERD requires careful consideration of the primary symptom presentation, degree of mucosal injury, and the presence or absence of complications. Treatment revolves around 4 goals: elimination of symptoms, healing of mucosal injury if present, management of complications, and maintenance of symptomatic remission. Treatment should combine lifestyle modifications, pharmacologic therapy, and appropriate use of antireflux surgery. GERD may recur quickly if therapy is stopped or medication dosage is decreased; therefore, long-term therapy is the key to effective management and often requires continuous full prescription doses of appropriate medications. Symptom relief and mucosal healing in GERD are directly related to control of intragastric acid secretion (time gastric pH <4) and reduction of esophageal acid exposure.[1] Clinical trials in patients with symptomatic erosive esophagitis suggest that a careful and systematic stepwise approach to medical therapy will result in satisfactory symptom relief in over 90% of patients.[1]

In contrast, there have been few clinical trials of treatment involving patients with asthma, cough, laryngopharyngeal reflux (LPR), and other extra-esophageal manifestations of GERD. Most are uncontrolled and maintenance trials are lacking. Treatment is based on the principles for testing patients with heartburn and erosive esophagitis or observations from available clinical trials and clinical experience. As a general rule, patients with LPR and the other extra-esophageal manifestations of GERD require higher doses of pharmacologic therapy, usually with proton pump inhibitors twice daily, with longer periods of treatment needed to achieve complete relief of symptoms compared to patients with heartburn and erosive esophagitis. Although relief of symptoms, healing of mucosal injury, and maintenance of remission are still the primary goals, assessing these end-points is somewhat more difficult as the "gold standard" for diagnosis is not always clear. This chapter reviews the principles of the medical treatment of GERD with specific emphasis on LPR and other extra-esophageal manifestations of GERD.

LIFESTYLE MODIFICATION AND PATIENT EDUCATION

Simple and effective changes in lifestyle are crucial in controlling symptoms of GERD. Education about the recurring nature and chronicity of GERD and LPR is crucial to compliance with long-term medical management. Studies with overnight pH monitoring have shown a significant decrease in total esophageal acid exposure after elevation of the head of the bed 6 inches compared to sleeping flat.[2] A similar effect can be produced by placing a foam rubber wedge under the patient's mattress. A long (full length) wedge is preferable to tilt the whole mattress rather than bending it at the waist level. The use of pillows in lieu of a wedge or head-of-the-bed elevation cannot be recommended because bending of the waist and change in body position may paradoxically increase intra-abdominal pressure and increase reflux. In addition, if patients roll over on their stomachs while sleeping on pillows, bending backward may result in lower back pain, which may lead them to stop complying with instructions to elevate their torsos.

Elimination or decreasing of esophageal irritants from the diet will reduce symptoms. These agents include citrus juices, tomato products, coffee (both caffeinated and decaffeinated), and alcohol. Colas, tea, and other acidic fluids are often overlooked as potential esophageal irritants.[3] A high fat meal will increase postprandial reflux episodes in patients with GERD,[4] so a low-fat diet is recommended. Chocolate and other carminatives will lower LES pressure and increase reflux frequency,[5] as will onions, and should be eliminated from the diet (Table 7-1).

TABLE 7-1. *Lifestyle Modifications for Treatment of Gastroesophageal Reflux*

Elevation of head of bed (6 inches)—avoid waterbed
Dietary modifications
  1. Lower fat, higher protein
  2. Avoid specific irritants
    a. citrus juices
    b. tomato products
    c. coffee, tea
    d. alcohol
    e. colas
    f. onions
  3. No eating prior to sleeping (allow at least 2 hours)
  4. Avoid chocolate carminatives (lower LES* pressure)
Decrease or stop smoking
Avoid potentially harmful medications
  1. Affect LES pressure
    a. Anticholinergics
    b. Sedatives/tranquilizers
    c. Theophylline
    d. Prostaglandins
    e. Calcium channel blockers
  2. Potentially cause esophageal injury
    a. Potassium tablets
    b. Ferrous sulfate
    c. Antibiotics (gelatin capsules), eg, tetracycline
    d. NSAIDS, aspirin
    e. Alendronate

*LES = Lower esophageal sphincter.

Gastric distention provides the major stimulus for transient lower esophageal sphincter relaxation (TLESR), the most common abnormality responsible for individual reflux episodes.[6] Eating large, high-fat meals increases gastric distention and slows gastric emptying, probably increasing TLESRs. Going to sleep on a full stomach or lying down after a meal also creates a stimulus for TLESR and is likely to increase reflux. It is therefore critical to remind patients to avoid eating within 2 to 3 hours of sleep and to avoid recumbency after a meal.

Medications that decrease esophageal pressures and promote reflux include anticholinergics, sedatives or tranquilizers, tricyclic antidepressants, theophylline, nitrates, and calcium channel blocking agents.[7] Many other drugs are known to cause direct esophageal injury (pill-induced esophagitis). The most common are KCL (potassium) tablets, iron-sulfate, gelatin capsule antibiotics, nonsteroidal anti-inflammatory drugs (NSAIDS),[7] and alendronate (Fosamax).[8] These should be used with caution in patients with GERD. Though there is no direct evidence that these agents cause GERD, they can cause esophageal injury and may make mucosal injury from reflux more severe (Table 7-1). The effects of these agents vary from patient to patient. Experience suggests that none of these drugs greatly exacerbates GERD, so discontinuing a needed agent is usually not necessary, especially with concomitant use of proton pump inhibitors.

Smoking can decrease LES pressure and delay esophageal clearance, increasing reflux frequency and potentially mucosal injury. This is likely due to the effects of nicotine. Smoking may decrease the effect of H_2-receptor antagonists, especially at night (when reflux injury is more severe due to delayed esophageal clearance of refluxate); no effect of smoking on efficacy of proton pump inhibitors is known. Clearly smoking can be detrimental to overall health—exacerbation of GERD is no exception.

One study examined the effect of lifestyle modifications including raising the head of the bed 6 inches, eliminating meals before bedtime, and using antacids in the treatment of patients with respiratory symptoms and GERD. Outcomes were compared to using no antireflux measures for 2-month periods. In this study both esophageal and respiratory symptoms were reported to improve with lifestyle modifications compared to no antireflux therapy. However, no objective changes were noted in pulmonary function and endoscopy was not performed.[9] This suggests that the addition of the conservative measures outlined in Table 7-1 are useful in treatment of extraesophageal GERD. No studies have specifically examined lifestyle modifications in patients with LPR. However, we routinely recommend their use, as patients often reflux in the postprandial period, even when upright.[10]

The importance of including lifestyle modifications as part of a treatment program at a time when very efficacious drug therapy, such as proton pump inhibitors, is available has been debated. All clinical trials have included these lifestyle changes as part of treatment, so the effect of eliminating them is not known. These interventions are easy to explain and implement and are of low economic cost. Based on symptom severity and control, patients can decide for themselves, how diligent they should be. Some patients with mild, infrequent symptoms may avoid regular prescription medications by following these recommendations. They appear somewhat less likely to be sufficient in many voice professionals, especially in singers who experience upright reflux when they sing due to increased intra-abdominal pressure that occurs with proper voice support.

OVER-THE-COUNTER AGENTS

Numerous antacids and over-the-counter H_2-receptor antagonists are available to treat patients with symptomatic reflux. These agents should be used exclusively to treat symptoms such as heartburn that is intermittent and as adjuncts to prescription therapy for breakthrough symptoms. Symptom relief is similar with equipotent antacids and all of the H_2-antagonists available over the counter. Because patients with LPR often require long-term (or lifetime) therapy with high doses of proton pump inhibitors or H_2-blockers in full prescription doses, there is rarely any place in their management for over-the-counter (low dose) H_2-blockers. The use of antacids remains controversial. Experts agree that they should be superfluous if *sufficient* doses of acid suppression therapy is used. However, there are differences of opinion regarding the level of control achieved in most patients on the customary doses (omeprazole 40 mg daily, or the equivalent), and on the importance of occasional episodes of breakthrough reflux. It is well known that reflux may occur on 40 mg of omeprazole or 60 mg of lansoprazole. This can be confirmed by pH monitor studies; and some patients require higher doses for complete acid suppression. The occasional reflux episodes experienced by many patients on 40 mg of omeprazole per day may be "normal" and not significant; however, in patients with LPR, especially voice professionals any laryngeal acid exposure is detrimental. Rather than doing 24-hour pH studies on medication for every patient with LPR, or prescribing even higher doses of proton pump inhibitors routinely, some physicians use antacids in addition to proton pump inhibitors. The antacids are used at bedtime and before strenuous exercise (such as singing). This regimen may be useful for singers whose laryngeal appearance improves but incompletely on proton pump inhibitors. Indeed, one might speculate that there could be a theoretical safety advantage to nearly complete acid suppression with supplemental antacids over profound suppression in young adults who may be treated for decades. Clearly, research into these important questions is needed.

H_2-RECEPTOR ANTAGONISTS

Since their introduction in the late 1970s H_2-receptor antagonists have been the mainstay of the treatment of GERD. The only mechanism of action of these drugs is to inhibit gastric acid secretion; they have no effect on LES pressure or esophageal clearance. The 4 available agents (cimetidine, ranitidine, famotidine, and nizatidine) are equal in efficacy when used in equivalent doses. These agents are extremely well tolerated in all age groups and achieve complete relief of heartburn in 60% of patients treated.[11] Healing of mucosal abnormalities in the esophagus is less frequent and often overestimated, being seen in 0% to 82% (mean 48%) of patients.[11] The best results are seen in patients with nonerosive esophagitis where success rates are as high as 75%.[11] Higher doses of H_2-antagonists, up to 4 times daily, are usually needed to treat erosive esophagitis[12]; however, the cost of this double-dose therapy is greater and therapy is not as clinically effective as using a single daily dose of proton pump inhibitors. Maintenance of heartburn relief and healing of esophageal mucosal injury is seen in only 25% to 50% of patients treated with full dose (eg, ranitidine 150 mg twice daily) continuous therapy of H_2-antagonist for 1 year.[13]

H_2-receptor antagonists are remarkably safe agents. Side effects are rarely seen with greater frequency than placebo in clinical trials. Rare cases of hepatitis, qualitative platelet defects, and mental confusion with intravenous use have been reported. Drug interactions are extremely rare, although they seem to be slightly more prevalent with cimetidine. Caution should be exercised in patients on dilantin, warfarin, and theophylline, although clinical problems are rare.[14] Cimetidine has also been associated with male infertility, a side effect that has not currently been seen with the other H_2-antagonists.

There are few trials in which H_2-receptor antagonists have been systematically evaluated in the treatment of extra-esophageal GERD; and all of the reported trials have been in patients with either asthma or chronic cough. The largest study by Larrain et al[15] randomized patients to placebo, cimetidine 300 mg 4 times a day, or antireflux surgery in a 6-month treatment trial. Most of the patients had mild GERD; before treatment heartburn was seen less than once a week in all patients and 66% had no evidence of esophagitis by endoscopic examination. All patients had abnormal esophageal acid exposure during prolonged pH monitoring. Both pulmonary and esophageal symptoms were improved in the cimetidine and surgery group compared to placebo. However, the response to surgical therapy was statistically superior to medical therapy. Response was slower than in typical patients with heartburn, with many patients achieving optimal response only after 4 to 6 months of treatment.[15] Another study comparing ranitidine, 150 mg 3 times daily, with antireflux surgery showed a statistical advantage for antireflux surgery.[16] These studies reinforce that the superior control of esophageal acid exposure seen after antireflux surgery compared to that of H_2-blockers may be needed for optimal relief of pulmonary (and other extra-esophageal) symptoms. Several other short-term studies using H_2-receptor antagonists in doses from 150 mg ranitidine at bedtime up to 150 mg 3 times a day for periods of 1 to 8 weeks have consistently demonstrated improvement in heartburn. However, they demonstrate limited improvement in objective changes of pulmonary function and symptoms at the end of these 8-week trials.[17-19] Improvements in respiratory symptoms, if they occurred, lagged weeks behind esophageal symptoms. A clear history of reflux-associated asthma was the only predictive factor for improvement in respiratory symptoms. Clinical experience confirms these findings.

Cimetidine has been used successfully in unblinded and uncontrolled trials of patients with chronic cough associated with GER. Improvement of cough is reported in 70% to 100%.[20-23] Time to symptom improvement was quite prolonged, usually about 161 to 179 days. Patients with heartburn as the primary GERD symptom usually improve in 1 to 3 weeks. Despite reports of clinical improvement, no correlation was seen between clinical response and reduction in esophageal acid exposure by prolonged pH monitoring, which was performed at the end of the study. Although they were used extensively before the introduction of proton pump inhibitors, there are no formal studies in which H_2-receptor antagonists have been used to treat LPR. Currently we use them only in patients who are unable to tolerate proton pump inhibitors. If they are to be used, high-dose therapy is required, using a minimum of the equivalent of ranitidine, 150 mg 4 time a day (Table 7–2).

PROKINETIC AGENTS

Drugs that increase LES pressure, and accelerate esophageal clearance and gastric emptying are ideal agents to "correct" the pathogenic defects in GERD. Unfortunately the results seen with the two most commonly prescribed prokinetic agents, metoclopramide and cisapride, have been somewhat disappointing in treating GERD. Equal efficacy is seen with either agent. Heartburn relief can be achieved with cisapride in close to 60% of patients when 10 mg is given 4 times a day and is equal in efficacy compared with H_2-receptor antagonists.[24] Recent studies suggest that comparable heartburn relief can be achieved with 20 mg twice a day, a dose that will increase compliance.[25]

The central nervous system side effects of metoclopramide (drowsiness, irritability, extra-pyramidal effects) make its use problematic, particularly in the elderly and in voice professionals. Because cisapride does not cross the blood-brain barrier these side effects are not seen, so it has largely replaced metoclopramide as the prokinetic agent of choice. The major side effects of cisapride are diarrhea (about 10%) and nausea. Prolongation of the QT interval and development of ventricular arrhythmias may be seen in patients on cisapride who are concomitantly treated with macrolide antibiotics (eg, erythromycin) or

TABLE 7-2. Standard Medical Therapy of Gastroesophageal Reflux

Agents	Dosage
Promotility agents	
Metoclopramide	5–10 mg 4 times a day
Cisapride	10 mg 4 times a day
Acid suppressive agents	
H_2-receptor antagonists*	
Cimetidine	400 mg 2 times a day (nonerosive symptomatic disease)
	800 mg 2 times a day (erosive esophagitis)
Ranitidine	150 mg 2 times a day (nonerosive symptomatic disease)
	150 mg 4 times a day (erosive esophagitis)
Famotidine	20 mg 2 times a day (nonerosive symptomatic disease)
	40 mg 2 times a day (erosive esophagitis)
Nizatidine	150 mg 2 times a day (all forms of reflux disease)
Proton pump inhibitors†	
Omeprazole	20 mg a day (AM) acute and maintenance therapy
Lanzoprazole	30 mg a day (acute)
	15 mg a day (maintenance)

*Also available over the counter in reduced dose for medication as needed.
†Higher doses are required for treatment of extra-esophageal disease. See text.

antifungal agents.[26] Use of these drugs in combination should be avoided.

Cisapride's major use is in patients with mild or nonerosive esophagitis who have nocturnal heartburn. Superior symptom relief and healing in combination with H_2-receptor antagonists is seen when compared to either drug alone. However, cost and compliance issues with this combination offer no advantage over proton pump inhibitors.

Prokinetic agents have been used alone or in combination therapy with H_2-antagonists for treatment of cough, predominantly in children, but they have not been extensively studied in asthma and/or LPR. Improvement in cough was seen in 64.5% to 100% of patients in 2 uncontrolled studies.[27,28] Cisapride was studied in 22 infants aged 4 to 26 weeks with abnormal sleep pattern characterized by apneic episodes and associated GERD by pH monitoring,[29] as well as a group of 19 children aged 3 months to 10 years (mean 7 years) with either nocturnal cough, wheezing, or bronchitis, all of whom also had GERD by pH monitoring.[30] Apnea, night cough, and asthma symptoms were improved in 70% to 90%. Objectively, GER was decreased by pH monitoring after treatment. A third study evaluating cisapride in 27 children (mean age 6 years) with refractory asthma and GER by pH monitoring reported partial or complete improvement in respiratory symptoms in 80% after 3 months of treatment.[31]

A recent preliminary study by Khoury et al,[32] a double-blind controlled trial in 16 adult patients with pulmonary symptoms and GERD documented by ambulatory pH monitoring, compared cisapride, 10 mg 4 times a day, with placebo and showed significant improvement in FEV_1 and FVC in patients on cisapride compared to placebo. No improvement in objective assessment of esophageal acid exposure by ambulatory pH monitoring or in esophageal symptoms could be documented. Prokinetic agents have not been studied in patients with LPR.

PROTON PUMP INHIBITORS ARE THE MOST EFFECTIVE NONSURGICAL TREATMENT FOR GERD

Proton pump inhibitors (omeprazole and lansoprazole) inhibit the H^+K^+ ATPase enzyme that catalyzes the terminal step of acid secretion in the parietal cell. Profound acid inhibition is possible with these agents, resulting in improved symptom relief and healing of erosive disease. A single daily dose of either drug will produce a 67% to 95% (mean 83%) rate of symptom relief and healing of erosive esophagitis.[33,34] A large trial comparing omeprazole 20 mg daily to lansoprazole 30 mg daily showed comparable healing rates of over 85% after 8 weeks of therapy.[35] Successful complete symptom relief and healing of erosive esophagitis is seen in 85% of patients when continuous therapy is given over 1 year.[36] Continuous therapy is significantly superior to alternate day or weekend therapy and to H_2-receptor antagonists in the long-term treatment of GERD. Continuous therapy with omeprazole, 20 mg to 60 mg a day, has been shown to maintain complete symptom relief and healing for up to 5 years even in patients refractory to H_2-antagonists.[37] This study illustrates several key points: long-term remission is possible in up to 100% of patients if adequate doses of proton pump inhibitors are used; up to 30% of patients refractory to H_2-antagonists will require either twice daily or more frequent dosing of proton pump inhibitors; and most patients respond to stable doses of omeprazole long term without the development of tolerance. A preliminary report of continued follow-up of this same patient group shows continued success of omeprazole for 11 years. Relapse occurred in one patient per 9 years of treatment, with minimal side effects.[38]

Combination therapy with proton pump inhibitors and prokinetics (principally cisapride) is commonly used in clinical practice in patients who are difficult to manage. Unfortunately, no studies have shown a statistical advantage for combination therapy compared to increasing the dose of proton pump inhibitors. Proton pump inhibitors appear to have their best effect when given before a meal; and if more than a single dose is required, they should be given in split doses twice daily before breakfast and dinner.[39,40] Omission of breakfast will reduce the efficacy of the proton pump inhibitors.[41] If proton pump inhibitors are used in combination with antacids, the medications should be separated by about an hour with the antacids being taken about one-half hour after meals. If an H_2-antagonist is added, it should be given at bedtime.

There are clinical situations in which difficulty swallowing mandates alternative methods of administrating proton pump inhibitors. Multiple studies with omeprazole and 2 studies with lansoprazole have shown that proton pump inhibitors can be given to patients who are unable to ingest intact capsules by opening the capsule and flushing the intact granules with water, preparing a bicarbonate-based suspension, administering the capsules in apple or orange juice, or sprinkling the granules on applesauce or yogurt. The capsules should not be crushed.[42] Adequate control of intragastric pH has been demonstrated when omeprazole suspension is given via percutaneous gastrostomy, jejunostomy, or nasogastric tube. This is particularly useful in postoperative patients prone to aspiration, patients at risk for stress ulceration, or the patient on chronic enteral feeding via gastrostomy tube.

Proton pump inhibitors have an excellent safety profile with no side effects greater than placebo seen in clinical trials. The major side effects, headache and diarrhea, are quite rare. There has been concern about long-term safety of proton pump inhibitors because of their profound acid suppression. Current evidence suggests this fear is unjustified, as ample gastric acid is produced in a 24-hour period to allow for normal protein digestion, iron and calcium absorption, and to prevent bacterial overgrowth and maintain B_{12} absorption. The most important concern with long-term use of proton pump inhibitor is hyperplasia of enterochromaffinlike (ECL) cells and development of gastric carcinoid tumors because of hypersecretion of gastrin. As of this writing, there have been no reports of gastric carcinoid or any gastric malignancy with up to 11 years of omeprazole.[38] Hyperplasia of ECL cells is seen in $\leq 4\%$ of patients on proton pump inhibitors. A recent study suggested that patients on long-term omeprazole who were infected with *Helicobacter pylori* (*H. pylori*) developed atrophic gastritis (a proposed precursor of gastric adenocarcinoma) at a more rapid rate than patients who were not infected, prompting these authors to recommend screening and treatment of *H. pylori* in patients on long-term proton pump inhibitors.[43] A recent FDA panel determined that these data are insufficient to support this recommendation.[44] No specific laboratory monitoring—in particular serum gastrin—is required for patients on long-term proton pump inhibitors.

Several clinical trials have been conducted using proton pump inhibitors in patients with extra-esophageal symptoms, principally asthma and LPR. All of the trials have been conducted with omeprazole. Two short-term studies, one with omeprazole 20 mg once a day for 4 weeks[45] and the other with 20 mg twice daily for 6 weeks,[46] showed an improvement in pulmonary function tests on omeprazole compared to placebo. However, little change in bronchodilator use or asthma scores could be demonstrated. A longer trial by Boeree et al,[47] a randomized double-blind controlled trial in 36 patients comparing omeprazole 40 mg twice daily to placebo for 3 months, showed a reduction in nocturnal cough during treatment with omeprazole compared to placebo. However, objective changes in FEV_1 and other pulmonary function tests were not seen.[48] The study by Meier et al[46] using 20 mg omeprazole twice daily found that 6 of 11 patients who failed to improve on omeprazole also did not heal their esophagitis. This suggests that acid suppression was inadequate in these patients. The patients who did have control of their asthma also had healed their esophagitis, reinforcing the fact that adequate acid control can relieve pulmonary symptoms.

Important insights into treatment of patients with extraesophageal GERD come from a well-designed study by Harding et al[49] in which 30 patients with documented asthma and proven GERD by prolonged pH monitoring were treated with increasing doses of omeprazole beginning with 20 mg a day, increasing by 20 mg daily after every 8 weeks of treatment for 3 months or until esophageal acid exposure was reduced to "normal." Normalization of esophageal acid exposure resulted in improvement in pulmonary symptoms in 70% of patients. There are several important observations from this trial: 8 of 30 patients (28%) required more than 20 mg of omeprazole daily to normalize esophageal acid exposure; many patients required the entire 3-month period of treatment to achieve optimal symptom relief with improvement progressing continuously over the 3-month period; a favorable response to omeprazole was seen in patients who presented with frequent regurgitation (greater than once a week) and/or abnormal proximal acid exposure demonstrated by ambulatory pH monitoring (see chapter 5). The study emphasizes the importance of adequate esophageal acid control to achieve improvement in patients with extra-esophageal symptoms. Complete elimination of esophageal acid exposure is often necessary in patients with extraesophageal disease (including LPR) to effectively relieve symptoms. The author requires that esophageal pH be greater than 4 for 99% of time during prolonged pH monitoring while on proton pump inhibitor therapy before accepting that acid suppression is optimal. In selected cases, even that is not adequate in patients with LPR if the 1% period of reflux includes proximal acid exposure with persistent laryngeal symptoms and signs.

Karnel et al evaluated 16 patients with posterior laryngitis (LPR) who had failed to respond to initial treatment with conservative, lifestyle measures for a 6-week period, with omeprazole 40 mg daily for at least 6 weeks.[50] Laryngeal and esophageal symptom scores improved significantly at the end of 6 weeks compared to pre-omeprazole scores. Objective improvement compared to pretreatment values was also seen when the larynx was evaluated by a blinded investigator using videolaryngoscopy. Six patients had improvement in their laryngoscopic scores but not laryngeal symptom scores. Symptoms relapsed within 6 weeks in all patients after therapy was stopped. Poorer response was seen in patients with abnormal proximal esophageal acid exposure on ambulatory pH monitoring. It is reasonable to speculate that 40 mg a day of omeprazole was inadequate therapy for these patients and that they might have responded to higher doses or to a regimen combining other medications.

The same authors studied 182 patients with posterior laryngitis and at least one of the following symptoms: postnasal drip, persistent or recurrent sore throat, cough, or hoarseness.[51] Patients were treated sequentially with conservative lifestyle modifications for an initial period of 6 to 12 weeks followed by famotidine 20 mg at bedtime for 6 weeks. Omeprazole 20 mg at bedtime was given to nonresponders. Omeprazole was then increased in 20 mg increments every 6 weeks until 80 mg a day was reached. Laryngitis was characterized as mild if posterior laryngeal erythema was seen; moderate if marked erythema, secretions, and mucosal granularity were present; and severe if ulceration, granulation tissue, or hyperkeratosis were seen. Patients with mild symptoms and minimal laryngeal changes responded to conservative measures or famotidine, whereas patients with severe laryngitis required proton pump inhibitors.[50] These studies emphasize variability in response of patients with LPR, the need to treat for longer periods before seeing a response when disease is severe, the need for higher doses of proton pump inhibitors, and the rapid relapse of symptoms when therapy is discontinued, emphasizing that long-term treatment is often needed in patients with LPR.

Wo et al[52] studied 22 patients with posterior laryngitis felt to be secondary to GERD and diagnosed by indirect laryngoscopy, using an

8-week trial of omeprazole 40 mg at bedtime. Laryngeal symptoms improved in 67%. Increasing omeprazole to 40 mg twice a day in nonresponders did not improve response. Relapse was seen in 40% when omeprazole was stopped. There were no predictors of response, although nocturnal symptoms were more common in nonresponders. Perhaps this group had nocturnal acid breakthrough and continued to reflux despite high-dose proton pump inhibitor therapy. It is likely that results would have been improved if omeprazole were given twice daily (before breakfast and dinner), a treatment regimen that produces superior acid suppression to other modes of administration of this drug.[52] The response rate to omeprazole in this trial does, however, support empiric therapy for LPR.

Metz and colleagues studied 10 patients with endoscopic laryngitis who also had GERD diagnosed by abnormal ambulatory pH monitoring. They used 40 mg omeprazole as a single daily dose and found improvement in 7 of 10 (70%) patients at the end of 8 weeks.[53] Jaspersen and colleagues studied 34 patients with laryngeal symptoms, laryngoscopic changes of LPR and erosive esophagitis with omeprazole 20 mg a day for 4 weeks reporting improvement in esophagitis and laryngeal symptoms 32 of 34 patients (92%). No comment was made about laryngeal examinations.[54] The latter 3 studies were uncontrolled but showed excellent results with omeprazole. Although lansoprazole has not been studied in this patient population, comparable healing rates for omeprazole 20 mg and lansoprazole 30 mg a day, respectively, are seen in erosive esophagitis,[35] suggesting that this proton pump inhibitor should be equally effective in patients with LPR and other extra-esophageal disease.

Suggested Approach to Treatment of LPR

Current practice suggests that proton pump inhibitor therapy is the treatment of choice for patients with LPR. A starting dose of omeprazole 20 mg twice daily, before breakfast and dinner, or lansoprazole 30 mg twice daily given in similar fashion, for 2 to 3 months is our initial minimum treatment trial. Current experience suggests that 70% of patients will respond to this therapy, although many will require longer treatment periods to achieve optimal results. One of the authors of this textbook (RTS) routinely also uses antacids 4 times daily for the first 3 to 4 weeks, then decreases the frequency, depending on laryngeal symptoms and signs. Formal studies have not been done yet to confirm clinical impressions, but anecdotally this approach works well with most patients remaining on antacids at bedtime and prior to exercise and a few patients needing more than 20 mg of omeprazole or 30 mg of lansoprazole twice daily.

Patients who have a good initial response to this therapeutic trial should be continued at the same dose for an additional 4- to 8-week period to assess continued improvement. If complete symptom relief and mucosal healing are not achieved at this point, the patient should be reevaluated with prolonged ambulatory pH monitoring studies while on therapy with proton pump inhibitor (see chapter 5) to assess the adequacy of intragastric acid suppression and elimination of distal and proximal esophageal acid exposure. If acid suppression is incomplete, additional medical therapy is indicated prior to assuming that the patient is a medical failure. If the patient has a poor response to the initial therapeutic trial, prolonged ambulatory pH monitoring should be performed while on therapy to evaluate drug efficacy.

Recent studies from our laboratory have shown that 70% of patients with GERD treated with twice-daily proton pump inhibitor therapy will continue to have gastric acid breakthrough (pH <4) for at least 1 hour in the overnight period.[55] Reflux will occur in 30% to 50% of these patients during this breakthrough period.[56] Another study from our laboratory found that 30% of patients with extra-esophageal reflux (asthma, cough, LPR) continue to have abnormal acid exposure (GER) despite therapy with twice daily proton pump inhibitor.[57] These patients require more aggressive medical therapy, as even small amounts of acid exposure may be injurious to the mucosa of the larynx oral cavity and airways. Doubling the dose of proton pump inhibitor (eg, omeprazole 40 mg twice daily) may be sufficient to effectively control esophageal acid exposure. However, some patients will have continued nocturnal gastric acid breakthrough and esophageal reflux despite high-dose proton pump inhibitor and may require the addition of an H_2-receptor antagonist to achieve optimal acid suppression.[58] Referral to a gastroenterologist for ambulatory pH monitoring to document the effectiveness of therapy and assess the presence of continued nocturnal acid exposure is indicated if patients are refractory to proton pump inhibitors.

The high prevalence of esophageal motility abnormalities, principally ineffective esophageal motility (distal esophageal contraction amplitudes less than 30 mm Hg in $\geq$30% of wet swallows)[58,59] in patients with extra-esophageal GERD suggests that adding a prokinetic agent to therapy with a proton pump inhibitor should be efficacious in treating these patients. Unfortunately, there are no published data comparing combination therapy (proton pump inhibitors plus cisapride or metoclopramide) with either twice-daily or higher doses of proton pump inhibitor alone. Although improvement of respiratory symptoms in patients with GERD has been demonstrated in a preliminary study with cisapride, no effect on esophageal clearance, no improvement in motility abnormalities, and no change in reflux frequency can be documented in these patients.[60] We do not routinely recommend adding a prokinetic agent to proton pump inhibitors. We reserve prokinetic agents for patients in whom adequate acid exposure cannot be accomplished with acid suppressive agents and for the patient with documented delayed gastric emptying.

Clinical experience suggests that most patients with LPR will have chronic GERD and will require long-term medical therapy and or consideration of antireflux surgery (see chapter 8) for long-term control. The dose of proton pump inhibitor and other medications and the decision to perform antireflux surgery should be individualized to maintain symptom relief and mucosal healing. Current evidence suggests that long-term medical therapy is safe and tolerance or tachyphylaxis is extremely rare. Patients who choose long-term medical therapy can be confident of excellent long-term control of acid-induced mucosal injury without worry of serious complications. Although comparison studies are not available, it is likely that long-term medical therapy with proton pump inhibitors and antireflux surgery are equal options for most patients with regard to acid injury; and the choice can be left to the patients in consultation with their treating physicians. Acid suppression does not always provide adequate control of symptoms in patients who note symptoms from suspected pH neutral or alkaline reflux, especially singers; although this cannot be documented by clinical trials, such patients may be considered for surgery.

REFERENCES

1. Bell NJV, Burget DL, Howden CW, et al. Appropriate acid suppression for the management of gastro-esophageal reflux disease. *Digestion*. 1992;51 (suppl 1):59–67.
2. Johnson LF, De Meester TR. Evaluation of the head of the bed, bethanecol, and antacid foam tablets on gastroesophageal reflux. *Dig Dis Sci*. 1981; 26:673.
3. Richter JE, Castell DO. Drugs, foods, and other substances in the cause and treatment of reflux esophagitis. *Med Clin North Am*. 1981;65:1223.
4. Becker DJ, Sinclair J, Castell DO, Wu WC. A comparison of high and low fat meals on postprandial esophageal acid exposure. *Am J Gastroenterol*. 1989; 84:782.
5. Wright LE, Castell DO. The adverse effect of chocolate on lower esophageal sphincter pressure. *Dig Dis*. 1975;20:703.
6. Dent J, Dodds WJ, Friedman RH, et al. Mechanism of gastroesophageal reflux in recumbent asymptomatic human subjects. *J Clin Invest*. 1980;65: 256–267.

7. Kikendall, JW. Pill-induced esophageal injury: case reports and review of the medical literature. *Dig Dis Sci.* 1983;28:174–185.
8. Dent J, Dodds WJ, Friedman RH, et al. Mechanism of gastroesopohageal reflux in recumbent asymptomatic human subjects. *J Clin Invest.* 1980; 65:256–267.
9. Kjellen G, Tibbling L, Wranne B. Effect of conservative treatment of oesophageal dysfunction in bronchial asthma. *Eur J Respir Dis.* 1981;62: 190–197.
10. Katz PO. Ambulatory esophageal and hypopharyngeal pH monitoring in patients with hoarseness. *Am J Gastroenterol.* 1990;85:38–40.
11. Sontag S, Robinson M, McCallum RW, et al. Ranitidine therapy for gastroesophageal reflux disease. Results of a large double blind trial. *Arch Intern Med.* 1987;147:1485–1491.
12. Euler AR, Murdocck RH, Wilson TH, et al. Ranitidine is effective therapy for erosive esophagitis. *Am J Gastroenterol.* 1992;88:520–524.
13. Vignieri S, Termini R, Leandro G, et al. A comparison of five maintenance therapies for reflux esophagitis. *N Engl J Med.* 1995;333:1106–1110.
14. Feldman M, Burton ME. Histamine$_2$-receptor antagonists: standard therapy for acid-peptic diseases. *N Engl J Med.* 1990;323:1672,1749.
15. Larrain A, Carrasco E, Galleguillos F, et al. Medical and surgical treatment of non-allergic asthma associated with gastroesophageal reflux. *Chest.* 1991;99:1330–1335.
16. Sontag SJ, O'Connell SA, Greenlee HB, Schnell TG, et al. Is gastroesophageal reflux a factor in some asthmatics? *Am J Gastroenterol.* 1987;82: 119–126.
17. Harper PC, Bergner A, Kaye MD. Antireflux treatment for asthma: improvement in patients with associated gastroesophageal reflux. *Arch Intern Med.* 1987;147:56–60.
18. Ekstrom T, Lindgren BR, Tibbling L. Effects of ranitidine treatment on patients with asthma and a history of gastro-oesophageal reflux: a double blind crossover study. *Thorax.* 1989;44:19–23.
19. Gustafsson PM, Kjellman N-IM, Tibbling L. A trial of ranitidine in asthmatic children and adolescents with or without pathological gastroesophageal reflux. *Eur Respir J.* 1992;5:201–206.
20. Irwin RS, Curley FJ, French CL. Chronic cough: the spectrum and frequency of causes, key components of the diagnostic evaluation, and outcome of specific therapy. *Am Rev Respir Dis.* 1990;141:640–647.
21. Irwin RS, Azwacki JK, Curley FJ, French CL, Hoffman PJ. Chronic cough as the sole presenting manifestation of gastroesophageal reflux. *Am Rev Respir Dis.* 1989;140:1294–1300.
22. Fitzgerald JM, Allen CJ, Craven MA, Newhouse MT. Chronic cough and gastroesophageal reflux. *Can Med Assoc J.* 1989;140:520–524.
23. Waring JP, Lacayo L, Hunter J, Katz E, Suwak B. Chronic cough and hoarseness in patients with severe gastroesophageal reflux disease. Diagnosis and response to therapy. *Dig Dis Sci.* 1995;40:1093–1097.
24. Blum AL, Adami B, Bouzo M, et al. Effect of cisapride on relapse of esophagitis. *Dig Dis Sci.* 1993;38:551–560.

25. Castell D, Sigmund C, Patterson D, et al. Cisapride 20 mg bid provides effective daytime and nighttime relief in patients with symptoms of chronic gastroesphageal reflux disease. *Am J Gastroenterol.* 1998;93:547–552.
26. Wiseman LR, Faulds D. Cisapride: an updated review of its pharmacology and therapeutic efficacy as a prokinetic agent in gastrointestinal motility disorders. *Drugs.* 1994;47:116.
27. Dordal MT, Baltazar MA, Roca I, Marques L, Server MT, Botoy J. Nocturnal spasmodic cough in the infant: evolution after antireflux treatment. *Allerg Immunol.* 1994;26:53–58.
28. Font C, Molkhou P, Petrovic N, Fraitag B. Treatment using motilium of gastroesophageal reflux associated with respiratory manifestations in children. *Ann Pediatr.* 1989;36:148–150.
29. Ekstrom T, Tibbling T. Esophgeal acid perfusion, airway function and symptoms in asthmatic patients with marked bronchial hyperactivity. *Chest.* 1989;96:995–998.
30. Smyrnios NA, Irwin RS, Curley FJ. Chronic cough with a history of excessive sputum production. *Chest.* 1995;108:991–997.
31. Ing AJ, Ngu MC, Breslin ABX. Chronic persistent cough and gastroesophageal reflux. *Thorax.* 1991;46:479–483.
32. Khoury R, Paoletti V, Cohn J, Gideon M, Bracy N, Katz PO, Castell DO. Cisapride improves pulmonary function tests in patients with gastroesophageal (GE) reflux and chronic respiratory symptoms. *Gastroenterology.* 1998;114:712.
33. Sandmark S, Carlsson R, Falso O, Lundell L. Omeprazole or ranitidine in the treatment of reflux esophagitis. *Scand J Gastroenterol.* 1988;23:625–632.
34. Hetzel D, Dent J, Reed W, et al. Healing and relapse of severe peptic esophagitis after treatment with omeprazole. *Gastroenterology.* 1988;95:903–912.
35. Castell DO, Richter JE, Robinson M, et al. Efficacy and safety of lansoprazole in the treatment of erosive esophagitis. *Am J Gastroenterol.* 1996;91:1749–1758.
36. Vignieri S, Termini R, Leandro G, et al. A comparison of five maintenance therapies for reflux esophagitis. *N Engl J Med.* 1995;333:1106–1110.
37. Klinkenberg-Knol E, Festen H, Jansen J, et al. Long term treatment with omeprazole for refractory esophagitis. *Ann Intern Med.* 1994;121:161-167.
38. Klinkenberg-Knol E. Eleven years' experience of continuous maintenance treatment with omeprazole in GERD-patients [abstract 180]. *Gastroenterology.* 1991;98:114.
39. Kuo B, Castell DO. Optimal dosing of omeprazole 40 mg daily: effects on gastric and esophageal pH and serum gastrin in healthy controls. *Am J Gastroenterol.* 1996;91:1532–1538.
40. Hatlebakk JG, Katz PO, Kuo B, Castell DO. Nocturnal gastric acid breakthrough with omeprazole 40 mg MG daily: does dosing schedule make a difference? *Gastroenterology.* 1998;114:591.
41. Hatlebakk JG, Katz PO, Castell DO. Proton pump inhibitors should be taken with meals for optimal control of gastric acidity. *Gastroenterology.* 1998;114:592.

42. Zimmerman A, Walters JK, Katona B, Souney P. Alternative methods of proton pump inhibitor administration. *Consultant Pharmacist.* 1886;19: 990–998.
43. Kuipers EJ, Lundell L, Klinkenberg-Knol EC, et al. Atrophic gastritis and *Helicobacter pylori* infection in patients with reflux esophagitis treated with omeprazole or fundoplication. *N Engl J Med.* 1996;334:1018–1022.
44. Proton pump inhibitor relabeling for cancer risk not warranted. *FDA Reports,* Nov. 11, 1996.
45. Ford GA, Oliver PS, Prior JS, et al. Omeprazole in the treatment of asthmatics with nocturnal symptoms and gastroesophageal reflux: a placebo-controlled cross-over study. *Postgrad Med J.* 1994;70:350–354.
46. Meier JH, McNally PR, Punja M, et al. Does omeprazole (Prilosec) improve respiratory function in asthmatics with gastroesophageal reflux? *Dig Dis Sci.* 1994;39:2127–2133.
47. Boeree MJ, Peters FTM, Postma DS, Kleiberbeuker JH. Effect of high dose omeprazole on airway hyperresponsiveness and pulmonary function in patients with obstructive lung disease. *Gastroenterology.* 1995;108:A61.
48. Klinkenberg-Knol EC, Meuwissen SGM. Combined gastric and oesophageal 24-hr monitoring and oesophageal manometry in patients with reflux disease, resistant to treatment with omeprazole. *Alimet Pharmacol Ther.* 1990;4:485–490.
49. Harding SM, Richter JE, Guzzo MR, et al. Asthma and gastroesophageal reflux: acid suppression therapy improves asthma outcome. *Am J Med.* 1996;100:395–405.
50. Jacob P, Kahrilas PJ, Herzon G. Proximal pH-manometry in patients with "reflux laryngitis." *Gastroenterology.* 1991;100:305–310.
51. Hanson DG, Karnel PL, Kahrilas PJ. Outcomes of antireflux therapy for the treatment of chronic laryngitis. *Ann Otol Rhinol Laryngol.* 1995;104: 550–555.
52. Wo JM, Grist WJ, Gussack G, et al. Empiric trial of high dose omeprazole in patients with posterior laryngitis. *Am J Gastroenterol.* 1997;92:2160–2165.
53. Metz DC, Childs ML, Ruiz C, Weinstein GS. Pilot study of the oral omeprazole test for reflux laryngitis. *Otolaryngol Head Neck Surg.* 1997;116:41–46.
54. Jaspersen D, Weber R, Draf W, Hammar C-H. Omeprazole for the treatment of reflux associated chronic laryngitis. *Gastroenterology.* 1996;110:A143.
55. Peghini PL, Katz PO, Bracy NA, Castell DO. Nocturnal recovery of gastric acid secretion with twice-daily dosing of proton pump inhibitors. *Am J Gastroenterol.* 1998;93:763–767.
56. Anderson C, Katz PO, Khoury R, Castell DO. Distal esophageal reflux accompanies nocturnal gastric acid breakthrough in patients with gastroesophageal reflux disease (GERD) on proton pump inhibitor (PPI) BID. *Gastroenterology.* 1998;114:229.
57. Katzka DA, Paoletti V, Leite L, Castell DO. Prolonged ambulatory pH monitoring in patients with persistent GERD symptoms. Testing while on therapy identifies need for more aggressive antireflux therapy. *Am J Gastroenterol.* 1996;91:2110–2113.
58. Peghini P, Katz P, Castell D. Bedtime rantidine decreases gastric and secretion and eliminates esophageal acid exposure overnight in a patient with

Barrett's esophagus taking omeprazole, 20 mg BID. *Am J Gastroenterol.* 1997;92:1723.
59. Leite LP, Johnston BT, Barrett J, Castell JA, Castell DO. Ineffective esophageal motility (IEM): the primary finding in patients with nonspecific esophageal motility disorder. *Dig Dis Sci.* 1997;42:1859–1865.
60. Fouad YM, Khoury R, Hatlebakk JG, Katz PO, Castell DO. Ineffective esophageal motility (IEM) is more prevalent in reflux patients with respiratory symptoms. *Gastroenterology.* 1998;114:506.

CHAPTER

Surgical Therapy for Gastroesophageal Reflux Disease

The history of surgical therapy for the treatment of gastroesophageal reflux began with Phillip Allison who was the first to correlate the symptoms of a hiatal hernia with gastroesophageal reflux.[1] His repair, described in 1951, emphasized the need to place the gastroesophageal junction intra-abdominally to improve its function. This maneuver alone, however, was found to be associated with a high rate of symptom recurrence. More sophisticated attempts at securing the gastroesophageal junction below the diaphragm culminated with the posterior gastropexy described by Hill in 1967.[2] This operation is still in use, although it has largely been replaced by fundoplication.

Rudolph Nissen described his gastric fundic wrap in 1956, followed by a flurry of interest in surgical management for this disease.[3] However, over the past 2 decades, surgical treatment for reflux had become much less commonly utilized, owing to the introduction of more effective medical therapy, specifically H_2-blockers and proton pump inhibitors.

In 1991, the first reports of laparoscopic antireflux surgery were published.[4] Minimally invasive approaches to this disease made operations more acceptable to gastroenterologists and patients, leading to a resurgence in interest for surgical correction of GERD. Since the initial clinical reports in 1991, numerous studies have been published on the laparoscopic approach to antireflux surgery.[5-18]

Medical therapy is effective in controlling *acid* reflux in the majority of patients with GERD. However, while usually effective in controlling symptoms, medical therapy does not correct the mechanical abnormality that causes reflux. Patients often require long-term or indefinite courses of medications, as discontinuation frequently leads to recurrence of symptoms. In a series of 196 patients with severe esophagitis responsive to omeprazole, 82% developed recurrent erosions within 6 months after cessation of therapy.[19] Moreover, the consequences of long-term acid suppression are unknown.

Spechler et al[20] compared the outcome of medical versus surgical therapy for complicated GERD. Surgery was significantly more effective, resulting in greater patient satisfaction, higher lower esophageal sphincter (LES) pressures, lower grades of esophagitis, and lower levels of esophageal acid exposure. This study had an average 2-year follow-up, but was done without the use of proton pump inhibitors.

INDICATIONS FOR SURGICAL THERAPY

Indications for surgery include persistent symptomatology despite reasonable medical management and patient intolerance to medications. Surgery may also be an option for patients who are concerned about the consequences of long-term medical therapy. In patients whose symptom control requires continuous medical therapy, surgery is an important option. Patients with complicated gastroesophageal reflux disease, manifesting Barrett's metaplasia, stricture, or ulceration and those who require long-term therapy, should also be considered for surgery.

In the past, surgery for GERD was infrequently recommended due to the risks associated with abdominal surgery under general anesthesia, significant postoperative discomfort, and the recognition of substantial long-term complications such as dysphagia, "gas bloat," and others. Since the initial description of the operation by Rudolph Nissen in 1956, the operation has undergone significant modifications that have lessened the incidence of postoperative complications.[21] In addition, the introduction of the laparoscopic approach to antireflux surgery has minimized the postoperative discomfort and many of the risks. It has also shortened postoperative recuperation from 6 to 8 weeks to 2 to 3 weeks, allowing patients to return to normal activities in an acceptable period of time.

PREOPERATIVE EVALUATION

Thorough preoperative evaluation is essential to successful surgical management of GERD. Although the typical patient with this disorder has well recognized gastrointestinal symptoms, GERD may underlie certain cases of asthma and other respiratory diseases, laryngitis, chronic cough, and chest pain. In addition, other upper gastrointestinal conditions may present with symptoms similar to those seen with GERD. Thus, it is critical to firmly establish the diagnosis and to exclude other conditions.

Further goals of preoperative evaluation are to assess the anatomy and physiology of the swallowing mechanism and stomach.

Adequacy of esophageal motility and gastric emptying are important preoperative considerations, as disorders in either of these areas will affect the choice of a surgical procedure. It is also important to document complications of reflux, specifically the presence or absence of Barrett's metaplasia, ulceration, or stricture.

The preoperative evaluation should include the following:

1. A complete history and physical examination is especially important both to determine symptoms related to reflux and to exclude other conditions. Evaluation of the general medical status is also crucial.
2. Upper gastrointestinal endoscopy is important to exclude other lesions and to assess for the presence or absence of Barrett's metaplasia. Stricture and ulceration may also be seen. The presence or absence of *Helicobacter pylori* may be determined.
3. Roentgenographic barium contrast study of the upper gastrointestinal tract defines the anatomy of the esophagus and stomach, as well as the relationship of the gastroesophageal junction to the hiatus. The length of the esophagus is easily assessed. A foreshortened esophagus would significantly alter surgical management, as discussed below. The presence of a sliding or paraesophageal hernia can be assessed. In addition, other anatomic abnormalities of the esophagus and stomach can be identified, such as strictures, webs, masses, or diverticulae. Furthermore, this is a dynamic study allowing the radiologist to assess the motility of the esophagus and the emptying function of the stomach. Although reflux of barium is not always identified, the absence of this finding does not rule out the presence of reflux, demonstration of significant reflux of barium during this radiographic procedure is almost always considered abnormal.
4. Twenty-four hour pH monitoring is considered the most accurate test for documenting the presence of abnormal acid reflux. This is particularly useful in patients who present with atypical symptoms

such as asthma, chronic cough, hoarseness, chest pain, and others. This study quantifies the amount of abnormal reflux, its relationship to symptomatology, its presence in upright or supine positions, and the relationship of reflux episodes to time of day and specific activities. Although it is not strictly obligatory to obtain this study in patients with typical symptoms of reflux and evidence of reflux by other means (eg, endoscopic evidence of ulcerative esophagitis or Barrett's metaplasia), having this study is a useful baseline to help objectively assess postoperative results.
5. Esophageal manometry is obligatory in the preoperative evaluation of the patient with GERD. This essential study provides information regarding lower esophageal sphincter pressure, length, and relaxation. It also provides vital information regarding esophageal motility. Major motor abnormalities of the esophagus alter the choice of surgical procedure.
6. Other studies and evaluation include pulmonary function and comprehensive voice evaluations in selected patients. These are particularly valuable in patients presenting with atypical symptoms. An assessment of gastric emptying should also be performed. This information can be obtained from the upper GI series or from a gastric emptying study. It is important to document the status of gastric emptying prior to surgical intervention that occurs in the area of the vagal trunks, as there have been occasional reports of postoperative gastroparesis.

PATHOPHYSIOLOGY OF GASTROESOPHAGEAL REFLUX DISEASE AND SURGICAL CORRECTION

Gastroesophageal reflux disease results from a loss of competence of the antireflux barrier at the gastroesophageal (GE) junction. Improper functioning of the GE junction can be due to multiple factors, including transient inappropriate relaxations of the lower esophageal sphincter, primary hypotension of the lower esophageal sphincter, shortened lower esophageal sphincter length, shortened intra-abdominal segment of the lower esophageal sphincter, loss of a flap valve, and others such as delayed gastric emptying and abnormalities in esophageal clearance.[22] Incompetence of the gastroesophageal barrier is a mechanical defect that is amenable to surgical correction. To maximize competence at the gastroesophageal junction and minimize postsurgical complications, the proper antireflux operation should include the following:

1. Mobilization of the esophagus to restore intra-abdominal length.
2. Correction of the diaphragmatic defect.

3. The creation of a short, loose fundoplication around the distal esophagus just proximal to the gastroesophageal junction anchored to the esophagus for stability.

CURRENT OPERATIONS FOR CORRECTION OF GASTROESOPHAGEAL REFLUX DISEASE

Antireflux procedures can be classified into 2 groups: those that involve some form of fundoplication and those that do not. They can also be classified by surgical approach, specifically whether performed through the abdomen or through the chest.[23] Additionally, all of these operations can be done open or with minimally invasive techniques (laparoscopic and thoracoscopic approaches).

In selecting an antireflux operation, all preoperative information needs to be considered. Esophageal function and motility affect the choice of operation. When motility is normal, the Nissen fundoplication with a full 360° wrap is the operation of choice. Conversely, with major motility abnormalities, a partial fundoplication is usually preferable.

Second, the length of esophagus is important. Esophageal shortening should be treated with the addition of a gastroplasty. Third, the presence or absence of hypersecretion of gastric acid may play a role in choice of surgical procedure. An acid-reducing procedure such as a selective vagotomy may be considered in addition to the antireflux procedure. Fourth, the finding of significant gastroparesis preoperatively may prompt consideration of an additional gastric procedure such as a pyloroplasty at the time of antireflux repair.

SURGICAL REPAIRS INVOLVING FUNDOPLICATION

Nissen Fundoplication

In 1956, Rudolph Nissen described his 360° gastric fundic wrap. Since that time, modifications regarding the length and looseness of the wrap have been made, allowing the most effective antireflux procedure with minimal morbidity. Currently, this is the most popular antireflux procedure. The steps in performing fundoplication, which are similar whether the approach is open or laparoscopic, include:

1. Incision of the gastrohepatic omentum at the gastroesophageal junction to expose the esophagus and the diaphragmatic crura (Figs 8-1 and 8-2).

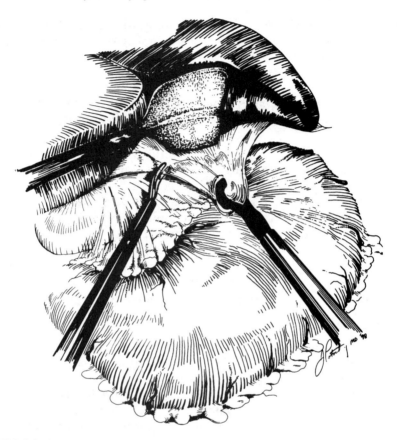

FIG 8-1. Incision of gastrohepatic omentum.

2. Identification and preservation of the anterior and posterior vagus nerves (Fig 8-3).
3. Circumferential dissection of the esophagus (Fig 8-4).
4. Assessment of mobility of the fundus.
    a. Mobilization of the fundus by division of the short gastric vessels if the fundus is not sufficiently floppy (Fig 8-5).
    b. With a sufficiently floppy fundus, mobilization of the short gastric vessels can occasionally be omitted, creating a Rossetti modification of the Nissen fundoplication.
5. Closure of the crura (Fig 8-6).
6. Construction of a loose fundoplication around the distal esophagus just proximal to the gastroesophageal junction. This is performed over a large (54-56 Fr) dilator and is created 2 cm in length (Fig 8-7).

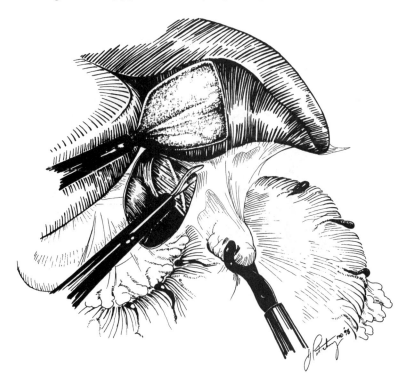

FIG 8-2. Exposure of esophagus and diaphragmatic crura.

The Laparoscopic Approach

In 1991 the first reports of laparoscopic antireflux surgery were published. These described a minimally invasive surgical approach to treatment of this disease with low mortality and morbidity. The laparoscopic approach can be used in most patients undergoing antireflux surgery and is becoming the approach of choice. Contraindications to a laparoscopic antireflux operation include major coagulopathy, severe obstructive pulmonary disease, and possibly pregnancy. Prior abdominal surgery is not a contraindication. Reoperative antireflux surgery usually cannot be performed laparoscopically. Occasionally, a laparoscopic approach may be attempted but conversion to an open procedure is necessary. This is usually due to severe central obesity or a large left lobe of the liver, both of which preclude adequate visualization of the relevant anatomy. The patient is placed on the operating table in lithotomy and reversed Trendelenburg positions. This allows the surgeon to be positioned between the patient's legs which facilitates

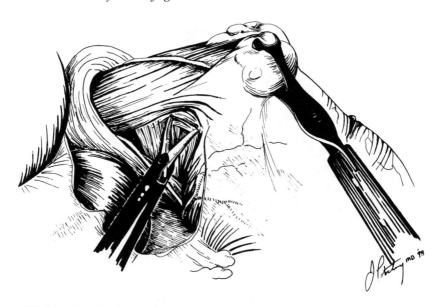

FIG 8-3. Identification of vagus nerves.

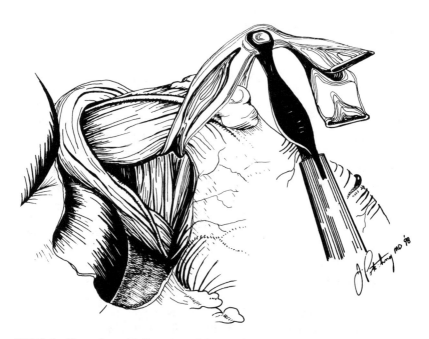

FIG 8-4. Circumferential dissection of the esophagus.

Surgical Therapy for Gastroesophageal Reflux Disease

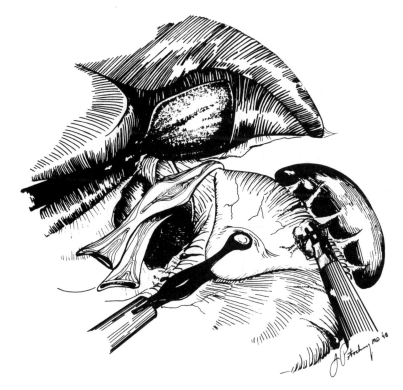

FIG 8-5. Mobilization of the proximal greater curvature.

2-handed dissection essential to satisfactory performance of this procedure. However, other reported surgical techniques suggest that the 2-handed technique can be used effectively with the patient in the supine position, having the surgeon on the left side of the table and modifying port placement somewhat (Fig 8-8).

A 12-mm port is positioned to the right of the xiphoid for the liver retractor. Right upper quadrant and left upper quadrant 10-mm ports are positioned, functioning as dissecting ports. An additional 10-mm port is placed in the midline for placement of the camera and a 10-mm port is placed in the left mid-abdomen for retraction of the stomach. The left lobe of the liver is retracted upward, exposing the gastroesophageal junction. A laparoscopic Babcock clamp is utilized to pull down on the fundus, exposing the hiatus.

The gastrohepatic omentum overlying the gastroesophageal junction is incised and the right crus is identified. The right crus is then dissected away from the right lateral wall of the esophagus. The left crus is then identified and dissected away from the left side of the esophagus. The esophagus is then retracted upward and the posterior aspect

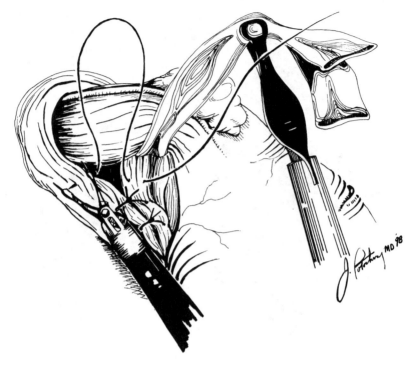

FIG 8-6. Closure of the crura.

of the esophagus is dissected under direct vision. It is important to perform the esophageal dissection under direct vision at all times to avoid perforation. Furthermore, dissection should not stray from the esophagus, as dissection into the pleural space can occur, causing pneumothorax. Once the esophagus is circumferentially dissected, a Penrose drain is placed around it and the Babcock previously used to retract the fundus is repositioned on the Penrose drain. The anterior (left) and posterior (right) vagus nerves are identified. The posterior nerve is excluded from the Penrose drain.

The fundus is then inspected to assess its mobility. In most cases, it is advisable to divide the short gastric vessels to allow for a loose, tension-free wrap. This can be accomplished using the harmonic scalpel or using clips. The proximal third of the greater curvature is mobilized in this manner.

The diaphragmatic opening is made appropriately snug. This is performed with a 54- to 56-Fr dilator within the esophagus to avoid making the closure too tight. Once the diaphragmatic closure is completed, the dilator is retracted into the mid-esophagus by the anesthesiologist. The fundus is then drawn around the posterior surface of the

Surgical Therapy for Gastroesophageal Reflux Disease

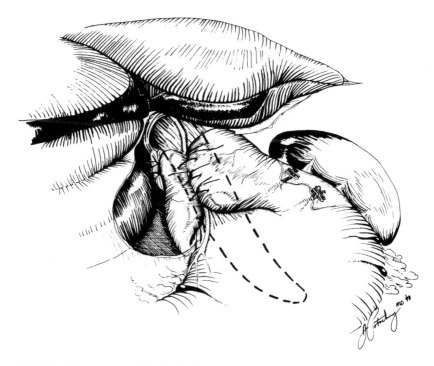

FIG 8-7. Construction of fundoplication.

esophagus. The wrap is accomplished over the 54-to 56-Fr dilator by placing three 2-0 silk sutures. These sutures are placed from the fundus to the esophagus to the other side of the fundus in each instance. The abdomen is then irrigated and hemostasis is ensured. All trocars are removed under direct vision and port sites are closed.

The Transthoracic Approach

Indications for performing an antireflux procedure via the thorax are:

1. Reoperative antireflux surgery.
2. Patients who require concomitant procedures on the intrathoracic esophagus.
3. Patients with coexistent left pulmonary pathology that needs surgery.
4. Patients with a foreshortened esophagus.
5. Obese patients in whom an abdominal approach may afford poor visualization.
6. Surgeon preference.

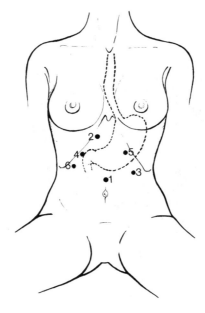

FIG 8-8. Port placement for laparoscopic fundoplication:
1. 30° laparoscope
2. Liver retractor
3. Stomach retractor
4. Dissecting port
5. Dissecting port
6. Optional dissecting port.

Partial Fundoplication

In the presence of esophageal dysmotility, partial fundoplication is the operation of choice. This can be performed through a thoracic approach such as a Belsey Mark IV partial fundoplication, which creates a 240° anterior partial fundoplication. Alternatively, the Toupet partial fundoplication can be performed transabdominally as an open or laparoscopic procedure. The technical aspects of this procedure are similar to those for the Nissen fundoplication with the exception of the wrap. After mobilization of the fundus and pulling it around posterior to the esophagus, the fundus is sutured to the right crus using three #2-0 silk sutures.

The anterior aspect of the fundus is then sutured to the esophagus. The fundus is similarly sutured to the left crus and anteriorly along the left side of the esophagus. This wrap necessitates placement of 12 sutures in the 4 rows (Fig 8-9).

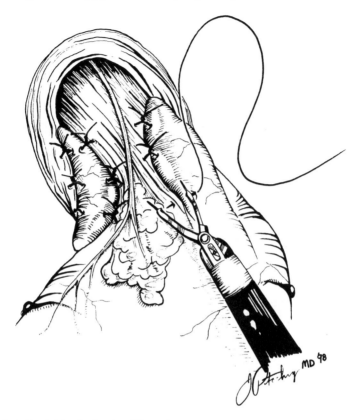

FIG 8-9. Partial fundoplication (Toupet).

Collis Gastroplasty

In patients with a foreshortened esophagus, a Collis gastroplasty is utilized to lengthen the esophagus. This is followed by a partial or complete fundoplication around the gastric tube with placement of the repair intra-abdominally (Fig 8-10).

NONFUNDOPLICATION REPAIRS (GASTROPEXY)

In 1967, Lucius Hill[2] described his experience with posterior gastropexy. After his initial series, approximately 20% of his patients had recurrence of reflux symptoms with long-term follow-up. This led to modifications of the technique to include calibration of the lower esophageal sphincter pressure intraoperatively. The physiologic basis of the current Hill

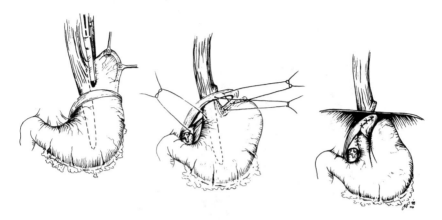

FIG 8-10. Collis gastroplasty.

operation is that the lower esophageal sphincter segment is restored to the high-pressure environment of the abdomen and secured in that position by anchoring the gastroesophageal junction to the median arctuate ligament posteriorly. The hiatal hernia defect is corrected, and the lower esophageal sphincter pressure is restored using intraoperative manometry (Fig 8-11).

The Hill repair has been described utilizing an open or laparoscopic technique.[24] The following steps are common to both:

1. The crura are dissected.
2. The anterior and posterior vagus nerves are identified and preserved.
3. The esophagus is dissected circumferentially.
4. The medial aspect of the gastric fundus is mobilized from its adhesions to the diaphragm, which occasionally also includes division of several short gastric vessels.
5. The preaortic fascia is dissected down to the area of median arctuate ligament.
6. The esophageal hiatus is loosely closed around the esophagus.
7. Sutures are placed in the anterior and posterior phreno-esophageal bundles, avoiding the esophagus. Three such sutures are placed.
8. Intraoperative manometry is performed. Sutures are placed through the imbricated bundles and carried through the preaortic fascia.
9. Additional sutures are placed from the fundus through the diaphragm to further reinforce the GE valve.

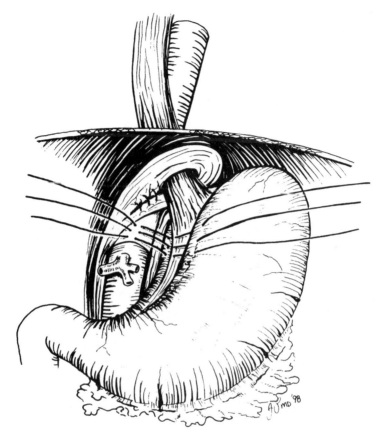

FIG 8-11. Hill posterior gastropexy.

POSTOPERATIVE CARE

Patients are admitted to the hospital postoperatively. A nasogastric tube is not used routinely. Antireflux medications are not restarted. On the first postoperative day, patients undergo an upper gastrointestinal contrast study using water-soluble contrast to rule out the presence of a leak. If no leak is identified, the patient is asked to swallow a small amount of barium to better delineate the postoperative anatomy and to assess emptying function of the esophagus and stomach. Clear liquids are started on the first postoperative day and diet is advanced as tolerated. With laparoscopic surgery, patients are generally discharged on the second postoperative day. Some degree of minor transient dysphagia is common, but in nearly all cases this resolves by 8 to 12 weeks.

Patients are seen in follow-up at 2 weeks. At 3 and 12 months, patients are asked to undergo repeat 24-hour pH monitoring and esophageal manometry.

OPERATIVE COMPLICATIONS

In general, antireflux surgery, whether performed open or closed, is safe. In several large series, mortality rates are essentially zero.[12,14] Wound complications such as infection and herniation are seen slightly more often with the open technique. In addition, splenic injury is reported as occurring in 1% to 2% of open fundoplications, but it is very rarely, if ever, seen with the laparoscopic approach.

Complications following laparoscopic antireflux surgery include those common to all operations, those specific to laparoscopy, and those related to the specific surgical procedure. Operative complications common to all procedures include bleeding and infection. Bleeding complications are rarely, if ever, seen with laparoscopic antireflux surgery. It is virtually never necessary to transfuse patients. Wound infection is also extremely uncommon. Another complication common to many operations performed under general anesthesia is pulmonary emboli. In our series of 70 laparoscopic antireflux procedures, this complication occurred in 2.8% percent of patients. In no instance was it fatal.[16]

Complications specific to laparoscopy include trocar injuries, hypercapnea requiring ventilation, pneumothorax, and pneumomediastinum. Trocar injuries are rare. We utilize an open technique for inserting the initial trocar and have not had any injuries. Many patients have pneumothorax. As part of the author's original protocol, all patients underwent routine chest X ray in the recovery room and this finding was incidentally noted commonly. In all instances, patients were asymptomatic, and the pneumothorax resolved on follow-up chest X ray the next day. In addition, pneumomediastinum with air occasionally tracking into the subcutaneous tissues of the neck and chest was also seen. In all instances, these findings resolved within 24 hours.

Complications specific to the operation include persistent dysphagia, defined as dysphagia still present more than 3 months after surgery. In the literature, patients have required reoperation for this complication, although we have not had that experience in our series to date. Occasionally, persistent dysphagia can be corrected with endoscopic dilatation. Postoperative gastroparesis is occasionally seen and thought to be due to edema around the vagus nerves secondary to the operative dissection. This complication is rare and is effectively treated with prokinetic agents such as Cisapride or Metoclopramide. This phenomenon is generally transient and these medications can be discontinued several weeks after surgery.

Esophageal or gastric perforation occurring intraoperatively has also been described. Should these complications be recognized intraoperatively, they can be repaired laparoscopically. However, this requires an experienced surgeon well versed in advanced laparoscopic techniques. Failure to recognize these complications may lead to septic complications, which frequently requires a return to the operating room. Fortunately, these are also rare.

RESULTS

Many studies report the efficacy of antireflux surgery with 90% of patients demonstrating symptom control. The laparoscopic approach achieves similar outcomes to open antireflux surgery, although follow-up is shorter.

Professional voice users will often demonstrate reflux during singing. This reflux may be acidic or pH neutral. This subgroup of patients does extremely well following surgery with improved vocal quality and strength.

SUMMARY

Antireflux surgery is a safe, effective therapeutic alternative in the management of gastroesophageal reflux disease. In expert hands, laparoscopic antireflux surgery is safe, effective, and corrects the underlying cause of reflux with minimal morbidity and high patient satisfaction. It eliminates the problems of pH neutral reflux and the need for prolonged use of acid-suppressing medications. Surgery should be considered as an appropriate option in the treatment of reflux disease.

REFERENCES

1. Allison PR. Reflux esophagitis, sliding hiatal hernia, and the anatomy of repair. *Surg Gynecol Obstet.* 1951;92:419–431.
2. Hill LD. An effective operation for hiatal hernia: an eight-year appraisal. *Ann Surg.* 1967;166;681–692.
3. Nissen R. Eine einfache Operation zur Beeinflussung der Refluxoesophagitis. *Schweiz Med Wochenschr.* 1956;86:590.
4. Geagea T. Laparoscopic Nissen's fundoplication preliminary report on ten cases. *Surg Endosc.* 1991;5:170–173.

5. Bittner HB, Meyers WC, Brazer SR, et al. Laparoscopic Nissen fundoplication: operative results and short-term follow-up. *Am J Surg.* 1994;167: 193–200.
6. Collet D, Cadiere GB. Conversions and complications of laparoscopic treatment of gastroesophageal reflux disease. *Am J Surg.* 1995;169:622–626.
7. Cuschieri A, Hunter J, Wolfe B, et al. Multicenter prospective evaluation of laparoscopic antireflux surgery. *Surg Endosc.* 1993;7:505–510.
8. Fontaumard E, Espalieu P, Boulez J. Laparoscopic Nissen-Rossetti fundoplication. *Surg Endosc.* 1995;9:869–873.
9. Geagea T. Laparoscopic Nissen-Rossetti fundoplication. *Surg Endosc.* 1994;8:1080–1084.
10. Hinder RA, Filipi CJ, Wetscher G, et al. Laparoscopic Nissen fundoplication is an effective treatment for gastroesophageal reflux disease. *Ann Surg.* 1994;200:472–483.
11. Jamieson GG, Watson DI, Britten-Jones R, et al. Laparoscopic Nissen fundoplication. *Ann Surg.* 1994;220:137–145.
12. McKernan JB, Laws HL. Laparoscopic Nissen fundoplication for the treatment of gastroesophageal reflux disease. *Am Surg.* 1994;60:87–93.
13. McKernan JB, Champion J. Laparoscopic anti-reflux surgery. *Am Surg.* 1995;6:530–536.
14. Peters JH, Heimbucher J, Kauer W, et al. Clinical and physiological comparison of laparoscopic and open Nissen fundoplication. *J Am Coll Surg.* 1995;180:385–393.
15. Rattner DW, Brooks DC. Patient satisfaction following laparoscopic and open antireflex surgery. *Arch Surg.* 1995;130:289–294.
16. Sataloff DM, Pursnani K, Hoyo S, Zayas F, Lieber C, Castell DO. An objective assessment of laparoscopic antireflux surgery. *Am J of Surg.* 1997; 174:63–67.
17. Snow LL, Weinstein LS, Hannon JK. Laparoscopic reconstruction of gastroesophageal anatomy for the treatment of reflux disease. *Surg Endosc.* 1995;9:774–780.
18. Weerts JM, Dallemagne B, Hamoir E, et al. Laparoscopic Nissen fundoplication detailed analysis of 132 patients. *Surg Laparosc Endosc.* 1993; 3:359–364.
19. Hetzel DJ, Dent J, Reed WD, et al. Healing and relapse of severe peptic esophagitis after treatment with omeprazole. *Gastroenterology.* 1988;95: 903–912.
20. Spechler SJ. Comparison of medical and surgical therapy for complicated gastroesophageal reflux disease in veterans. *New Eng J Med.* 1992;326: 786–792.
21. Rossetti M, Hell K. Fundoplication for the treatment of gastroesophageal reflux in hiatal hernia. *World J Surg.* 1977;1:439–444.
22. Hunter JG, Pellegrini CA, eds. Surgery of the esophagus. *Surg Clin North Am.* 1977;77:959–1217.
23. Skinner DB, Belsey RHR. *Management of Esophageal Disease.* Philadelphia, Pa: WB Saunders Co; 1988.
24. Hill LD, Kraemer SJM, Aye RW, Kozarek RA, Snopkowski P. Laparoscopic Hill repair. *Contemp Surg.* 1994;1:13-20.

Index

A
Abduction, 6
Achalasia, 34, 36
Adduction, 6
Air pressure, and fundamental frequency control, 15–17
Allison, Phillip, 89
Anatomy, of esophagus, 19–20
Antacids, 73
 for LPR, 81
Antireflux procedures, 93. *See also* Surgical therapy for GERD
Apnea, acid-induced, 49–50
Arytenoids, 6
Aspiration, 2, 62
Asthma. *See also* Gastroesophageal reflux disease, extraesophageal
 exercise-induced, 46
 expiration muscles, damage from, 11
 and H_2-blocker use, 74–75
 occurrence of, 37
 prokinetic agents for treatment, 76–77

B
Barium radiographs, 56–57
 for preoperative evaluation, 91
Barium swallows, 47
 with water siphonage, 57
Barrett's esophagus, 35, 36, 38
 assessing presence of, 91
Bed
 eating before, 43
 torso elevation in, 70
Belsey Mark IV partial Fundoplication, 100
Bilirubin pigment detection, 62–63
Body, 10
Botulinum toxin injection, 49
Brain, role in voice production, 11–12
Breathy phonation, 17
Bronchitis, as symptom of GERD, 37

C
Carcinoma, 49, 78–79
Central nervous system (CNS), involuntary response stimulation during swallowing, 21–22
Chest pain, unexplained, 36–37
Cholecystokinin, 29
Cimetidine, 73–75
Cisapride, 75–77
Collis gastroplasty, 101
Combination therapy, 78, 82–83
Conversational speech, infraglottic pressure for, 13
Cough, chronic, 37–38, 41
 prokinetic agents for treatment, 76–77
Cover, 10
Cricoarytenoid joint arthritis, 45
Cricothyroid muscle, 6

D
Deglutition. *See* Swallowing
Deglutitive inhibition, 24, 31–32

Dental enamel, loss of, 38, 42
Diagnosis of GERD, 55–65
Diaphragm, 11
Diet, modification of, 70
Drugs, reflux-promoting, 71–72
Duration response, 30
Dyspepsia, 34
Dysphagia, 64
　postoperative, 104–105
Dysphonia, from LPR, 2

E

Edema of mucosa, 42
Endoscopy, upper gastrointestinal, for preoperative evaluation, 91
Enterochromaffinlike (ECL) cells, hyperplasia from proton pump inhibitor use, 78–79
Erosive esophagitis, 35, 77
Erythema of mucosa, 42
Esophageal acid exposure
　detection of, 60–63, 65
　reduction of, with proton pump inhibitors, 79–80
Esophageal irritants, 70
Esophageal manometry, 63, 92
Esophageal motility abnormalities, 38
　and surgical therapy technique, 38, 92, 93
　treatment of, 82–83
Esophageal peristalsis, control of, 29–32
Esophageal smooth-muscle responses, in vitro, 30–31
Esophageal sphincters, 19, 20. *See also* Lower esophageal sphincter pressure
　importance of, 25–29
Esophageal stage of swallowing, 22, 24–25
Esophagitis, 38
　erosive, 35, 77
　pill-induced, 71
　progression of, 35
Esophagus
　anatomy of, 19–20
　innervation of, 19, 29–30
　length of, 93, 101

Evaluation, 46–47
　preoperative, 91–92
External intercostal muscles, 11
Extrinsic laryngeal muscles, 8

F

Famotidine, 73
Flow glottography, 17
Flow phonation, 17
Formants, 15
Frequency, 14
Fundamental frequency, 15–16
Fundoplication, 89, 93–101
　partial, 101

G

Gastric distension, 71
Gastric emptying, assessment of, 91–92
Gastric fundic wrap, 89
Gastric tumors, from proton pump inhibitor use, 78–79
Gastroenterologists, role in LPR management, 2
Gastroesophageal (GE) junction, improper functioning of, 92–93
Gastroesophageal reflux, prevention of by lower esophageal sphincter, 27, 29
Gastroesophageal reflux disease (GERD), 1
　chronicity of, 38–39
　complications of, 38, 57
　diagnostic tests for, 55–65
　medical treatment of, 70–83
　relapse in, 77, 90
　surgical therapy for, 3, 89–105
　symptoms, atypical, 36–38, 91–92
　symptoms, typical, 33–36
　treatment objectives, 69–70
Gastroesophageal reflux disease, extraesophageal, 36–38
　H_2-blockers for, 74–75
　proton pump inhibitors for, 79–80
Gastropexy, 101–102
Glottis, 6
Granulomas, laryngeal, 45–49

H

Heartburn, 33–35
  and atypical GERD symptoms, 37
  versus dyspepsia, 34
  H_2-blockers for, 74. See also
    H_2-blockers
  pH monitoring for, 61
  prokinetic agents for, 75–77
Hiatal hernia, 63–64
Hill, Lucius, 101
Hoarseness
  in morning, 41
  as symptom of GERD, 1, 37, 38
H_2-blockers, 50, 73–75
  effectiveness and use of, 2
  over-the-counter, 73
  side effects and drug interaction
    effects of, 74
  use on granulomas, 48
Hyperfunction, and reflux laryngitis, 42
Hypopharynx, probes in, 61

I

Ineffective esophageal motility (IEM),
  63
Infraglottic pressure, 13
Infraglottic vocal tract, 11
Intrinsic muscles of larynx, 6
Intubation granuloma, 45

L

Lamina propria, 10
Lansoprazole, 77. See also Proton
  pump inhibitors
Laparoscopic antireflux surgery, 3,
  89–90, 95–99
Laryngeal cartilages, 6–8
Laryngeal electromyography (EMG),
  43
Laryngeal granulomas, 44–49
  etiology of, 45
  evaluation of patients with,
    46–47
  recurrence of, 48–49
  surgery for, 48
  treatment of, 46–47
Laryngeal skeleton, 6–8
Laryngeal ulcers, 45
  etiology of, 45
  evaluation of patients with, 46–47
  surgery for, 48
  treatment of, 47
Laryngologists, role in LPR
  management, 2
Laryngopharyngeal reflux (LPR), 1.
  See also Gastroesophageal
  reflux disease,
    extraesophageal
  long-term medical therapy for, 83
  over-the-counter agents for, 73
  pathophysiology of, 43–50
  proton pump inhibitor therapy for,
    80–81
  structures affected by, 1–2
  symptoms of, 5
  treatment of, 47, 81–83
Larynx
  anatomy of, 5–10
  soft tissues of, 9–10
Latency gradient, 31
Lifestyle modifications, 70–72
  for LPR management, 47
Lower esophageal sphincter (LES), 20
  function of, 26–29
Lower esophageal sphincter pressure
  determining, with esophageal
    manometry, 63
  and hernias, relationship of, 63–64
  increasing, with prokinetic agents,
    75–77
  peptides and hormones, effects on,
    29
  resting, 27–29
Lower esophageal sphincter
  relaxation, 27
  as neural event, 27, 28

M

Manometry, 63, 92
Medical therapy, 2
  discontinuation of, and
    reoccurrence of symptoms, 90
  versus surgical therapy, 90
Medications
  for LPR, 47
  reflux-promoting, 71–72

Metoclopramide, side effects of, 75
Mirror examination, 46
Mucosa, 9–10
  acid exposure, effects on, 44–45
  erythema and edema of, 42
Mucosal wave, 14–15
Muscular tension dysphonia (MDT), 2
Myenteric (Auerbach) plexus, 30

N

Nasal cavity, 15
Neurolaryngology, 6
Neurotransmitters, effect on LES pressure, 27–29
Nissen fundoplication, 3, 63, 93–94
  Rosetti modification of, 94
Nissen, Rudolph, 89, 93
Nizatidine, 73
Nocturnal gastric acid breakthrough, treatment of, 82

O

Odynophagia, 38
Off-response, 30
Omeprazole, 47, 48, 77–81. *See also* Proton pump inhibitors
  resistance to, 50
  response to, 65
On-response, 30
Oral cavity, 15
Oral stage of swallowing, 21
Oral steroids, for granuloma treatment, 47
Oscillator, 6
Otolaryngologic abnormalities, management of, 64–65
Otolaryngologists, role in LPR management, 2, 3
Otolaryngology patients
  LPR management issues for, 2–3
  medical therapy for, 62
Over-the-counter medications, 73

P

Patient education, 70–72
Penrose drain, 98
Peptic strictures, 38

  detecting, in preoperative evaluation, 91
  and heartburn symptoms, 35
Peristalsis, 22–24
  esophageal, 29–32
  inhibition of, 24–25
pH monitoring
  limitations on, 64–65
  for LPR patients, 82
  during preoperative evaluation, 91–92
  prolonged, 60–63
pH-neutral or alkaline reflux, 50, 62–63
  and acid suppression, 83
Pharyngeal stage of swallowing, 21–22
Pharynx, 15
Phonation
  power source, oscillator, and resonator interaction, 13
  pressed, 17
Physical examination, 42–43
Physiology
  of esophagus, 21–32
  of voice, 11–17
Pitch, and frequency, 14
Posterior gastropexy, 89
Posterior glottic and supraglottic stenosis, 45
Posterior laryngitis, 44–50
Postoperative care, 103–104
Power source for voice, 11
Pregnancy, LES pressure during, 29, 43
Pressed phonation, 17
Primary peristalsis, 22
Professional Voice: The Science and Art of Clinical Care, 5
Professional voice users
  antacid use by, 73
  barium swallows with water siphonage for, 57
  chronic gastroesophageal reflux occurrence in, 1
  hyperfunctional technique use by, 42
  LPR occurrence in, 43
  LPR management issues for, 2–3

Prokinetic agents, 75–77
 and proton pump inhibitors,
  combination therapy, 78, 82–83
Proton pump inhibitors, 77–83
 administration techniques, 78
 effects of, 2, 47
 lack of response to, and pH
  monitoring, 62
 prior to and following surgery, 48
 and prokinetic agents, combination
  therapy, 78, 82–83
 safety profile of, 78–79
 therapeutic trial of, 56
 use of, 50
Pulmonologist, role in LPR
 management, 2
Pyrosis. *See also* Heartburn

R

Ranitidine, 73–75
Recurrent laryngeal nerves, 6
Reflux
 and granuloma, 47
 of pH-neutral or alkaline liquids,
  50, 62–63, 83
Reflux laryngitis (RL), 1
 and carcinoma, causal relationship
  of, 49
 physical examination for, 42–43
 and sudden infant death
  syndrome, 49–50
 symptoms of, 41–42
 and wound healing, delayed, 49
Regurgitation, 33–36
 and atypical GERD symptoms,
  association with, 37
 pH monitoring for, 61
Resonators, 11, 15
Respiratory muscles, 11
Roentgenographic barium contrast
 studies, 91

S

Science of the Singing Voice, The, 5
Secondary peristalsis, 22
Singer's formant, 15
Singers. *See also* Professional voice
  users

chronic gastroesophageal reflux
 occurrence in, 1
classically trained, 8
Singing, role of brain in, 12
Smoking, and LES pressure, 72
Sound of voice, 15
Speech-language pathologists
 assessment of patients with
  granulomas, 46–47
 role in LPR management, 2
Stomach, preoperative evaluation of,
 91–92
Stress, effects of, 43, 46
Strobovideolaryngoscopy, 43
 for granuloma or ulcer
  examination, 46
Subglottic pressure, 13–14
Subglottic stenosis, 45
Sudden infant death syndrome
 (SIDS), and RL, 49–50
Superior laryngeal nerve, 6
Support mechanism for voice, 11
Supraglottic vocal tract, 11
Surgical therapy for GERD, 89–105
 complications of, 104–105
 efficacy of, 105
 esophageal manometry prior to, 63
 fundoplication, 93–101
 GE junction correction, 92–93
 versus H_2-blockers, 74
 indications for, 90
 versus medical therapy, 90
 postoperative care, 103–104
 preoperative evaluation, 91–92
 technique selection, 93
Swallowing
 relaxation of LES during, 27
 and respiratory function,
  interaction of, 29
 stages of, 21–25
 and UES tone, 19

T

Tactile feedback, use of, 13
Tertiary contractions, 24
Therapeutic trial, 47, 55–56, 65
Therapy, long-term, 69
Thyroarytenoid muscle, 6

Toupet partial fundoplication, 63, 100
Transient lower esophageal sphincter relaxation (TLESR), 71
Transition, 10
Transthoracic antireflux surgery, 99–100
Treatment of GERD
   H_2-blockers for, 73–75
   lifestyle changes for, 70–72
   over-the-counter agents for, 73
   prokinetic agents for, 75–77
   proton pump inhibitors for, 77–83
Trocar injuries, 104

U

Upper esophageal sphincter (UES), 19
   function of, 25–26

V

Vagus nerve stimulation, and reflux, 44
Vocal folds, false, 6
Vocal folds, 6
   mechanical properties of, changing, 15–17
   movement of, during phonation, 13–14
   mucosa over, 10
   pathology of, 43–44
Vocal intensity, 17
Vocalis muscle, 6
Voice
   abnormalities, from reflux, 43–44
   analysis of, 43
   anatomy of, 5–11
   physiology of, 11–17
   source, 16
Voice rest, following surgery, 48
Voice team, 2
   assessment of granuloma by, 46–47
Voice warm-up, prolonged, 38, 41

W

Waterbrash, 34
Wound healing, delayed, 49